C0-AJQ-567

Parent-Child
Group Therapy

Parent-Child Group Therapy

Building Self-Esteem in a Cognitive-Behavioral Group

L. Eugene Arnold
The Ohio State University

Donna Estreicher
The Ohio State University

Lexington Books
D.C. Heath and Company/Lexington, Massachusetts/Toronto

218001

616.8915
A 756

Library of Congress Cataloging in Publication Data

Arnold, L. Eugene, 1936–
  Parent-child group therapy.

  Includes bibliographies and index.
  1. Group psychotherapy. 2. Family psychotherapy.
3. Cognitive therapy. I. Estreicher, Donna. II. Title.
RC488.A68   1985   616.89'156   84–40723
ISBN 0–669–09934–1 (alk. paper)

Copyright © 1985 by D.C. Heath and Company

All rights reserved. No part of this publication may be reproduced
or transmitted in any form or by any means, electronic or mechanical,
including photocopy, recording, or any information storage or retrieval
system, without permission in writing from the publisher.

Published simultaneously in Canada
Printed in the United States of America on acid-free paper
International Standard Book Number: 0–669–09934–1
Library of Congress Catalog Card Number: 84–40723

To our spouses and children, who helped us realize the subtleties of the parent-child relationship

Contents

Preface

T he treatment approach described in this book evolved out of clinical experience with behavior and learning disorders. This cluster of disorders includes the psychiatric diagnoses of attention deficit disorder (with or without hyperactivity), conduct disorder, and specific developmental disorders. The *Diagnostic and Statistical Manual, Third Edition* (DSM-III) acknowledges a large overlap among these three diagnostic categories, with many children manifesting two or even all three simultaneously. Common denominators include low self-esteem (self-image of failure, troublemaker, bad boy, or klutz), discouragement, failure to experience success, inability to achieve gratification by task completion, experiencing the world as an aversive paradigm, having disappointed, frustrated, or angry parents, and failure of rule-governed behavior. This last feature may manifest as difficulty applying a general rule to specific situations, difficulty acting on a rule, or difficulty utilizing other people's experience summarized in rules. So prevalent is it that Barkley has proposed making failure of rule-governed behavior a fourth criterion for diagnosis of attention deficit disorder (ADD) with hyperactivity (the first three being impulsiveness, inattentiveness, and hyperactivity).[1] These syndromes, in the aggregate, affect at least 10 percent of children at some point in their development. At least 3 percent suffer attention deficit disorder and 10 to 20 percent specific developmental disorders. Although prevalence estimates for conduct disorders are not readily available, they seem ubiquitous in clinical practice.

The disorders are so common among child psychiatry clinic patients that in 1976 the Ohio State University Child Psychiatry Clinic began experimenting with a group treatment format. The core of this treatment is a cognitive-behavioral approach[2,3] but with elements of reality therapy, sensory integration, insight, education, family systems, and parent guidance. Eventually it became clear that the new group format could be applied to many childhood problems besides behavior and learning disorders. The latter, however, have remained our main focus and provide most of the clinical examples in this book.

The need of disordered children for structure is recognized in the highly stylized, structured format described in the six chapters of part I. Part II illustrates clinical application with examples, transcripts, and specific discussion of techniques, tactics, and strategies. Part III, dealing with clinical training, presents examples of supervisory sessions.

Notes

1. Russell A. Barkley, "Guidelines for Defining Hyperactivity in Children," in *Advances in Clinical Child Psychology,* vol. 5, ed. B.B. Lahey and A.E. Kazdin (New York: Plenum Publishing Corp., 1982).

2. P.C. Kendall and L. Braswell, "Cognitive-Behavioral Self-Control Therapy for Children: A Components Analysis," *Journal of Consulting and Clinical Psychology 30 (1982:672–689:* Philip C. Kendall, ed. *Advances in Cognitive-Behavioral Research and Therapy* (New York: Academic Press, 1982), vol. 1; P.C. Kendall and S.D. Hollon, eds. *Cognitive-Behavioral Interventions: Theory, Research, and Procedures* (New York: Academic Press, 1979).

3. Donald H. Meichenbaum, *The Nature and Modification of Impulsive Children: Training Impulsive Children to Talk to Themselves.* Educational Resources Information Center, U.S. Office of Education Microfiche #ED073834, Apr. 10, 1971; Donald Meichenbaum, *Cognitive-Behavior Modification: an Integrative Approach* (New York: Plenum Press, 1977).

Acknowledgments

The parent-child group therapy format described in this book would not have been developed without the instigation of Katherine N. Dixon, M.D., who as chief of the Ohio State University Child and Adolescent Psychiatry Outpatient Clinic was bold enough to suggest that something constructive might come out of treating hyperkinetic children in a group. Essential contributions to the development of the group were made by Herman A. Tolbert, M.D., Hisako Koizumi, M.D., Elaine Nemzer, M.D., Mahendra Mahajan, M.D., and Marla Lake, M.D., during their respective tenures as outpatient chief resident. A breakthrough in the group's development was the introduction of sensorimotor activities by Katherine Sheridan, OTR. The book itself would not have been possible without the secretarial assistance of Theresa Niznansky and Dorothy Walker.

Part I
Group Format

1
Basic Format and Philosophy

Between four and eight (rarely nine) children and their parents meet weekly with at least three staff in a multifamily group. The term *multifamily* in this context does not mean that all members of each family are present. Siblings (and sometimes one of the parents) of the identified child patient are usually absent. On the other hand, grandparents, aunts, sitters, boyfriends or girlfriends of single parents, and even teachers and caseworkers, sometimes attend, so that each family usually averages about three people in attendance. Including staff, it is not unusual to have a group of two dozen people.

Most families are referred to the open-ended group after intake screening and evaluation in the child psychiatry clinic. For the first month they are expected to attend weekly, but gradually lengthen the intervals between groups attended as the child and situation improve. If necessary because of distance or parents' work schedule, a family may negotiate every-two-week attendance from the beginning. Most families attend about ten times over a three or four-month period, and this expectation is stated at entry, but a few continue more than six months. A few have even returned for a couple brush-up sessions a year or two later.

Structure and Mechanics

Sometimes the therapeutic modality described in this book is called sandwich multifamily group therapy because it is like a time sandwich. The first slice of bread is a session of ten to fifteen minutes with the parents and children together (first parent-child segment). The meat of the sandwich is a forty to fifty minute separate children's group. The cheese is a separate parents' group at the same time as the children's group. The final slice of bread is thirty to forty-five minutes with the children and parents back together again (final parent-child segment). The total sandwich takes about an hour and forty minutes, give or take 10 minutes.

Although the length of the group was not originally intended to be variable, this has proved a useful feature. It teaches the children (and parents) by modeling and experience to stick with a task until completion. Fatigue, boredom, whim, or running out of time are not accepted as excuses or reasons for noncompletion. The emphasis is on completion of each small task making up the various segments of the group, one by one, and the attention span is gradually extended minute by minute to the completion of the known tasks.

By the second or third time in attendance, most children have memorized the segments and sequence of the group and are reinforced for remembering them. They know after their first exposure to the group that they will be expected the next time to know what is done and the order in which it is done and will have a chance to experience success in reciting to the whole group on that topic. This is one of the first elements of the success experience to which they are intrusively and coercively exposed in the group.

Experiencing Success

Most of the children in the group have not previously been able to experience success at school and sometimes not on the athletic field or at home. Many have come to believe that they are hopeless; they have a failure self-image. The group format, structure, and techniques assume that the best antidote for a failure image is to experience success. Tasks are set up that are within the child's reach. Some of these success experiences are as simple as being able to answer a question about what comes next in the group. They range from being able to guess correctly the purpose of some activity, through being able to offer an opinion that is respected by the rest of the group, being able to guess what the group leader has in mind, being able to pick a reasonable assignment for the coming week and devise a creative plan for implementing it, to carrying out the homework project and reporting on its success at the following session.

Success is continually redefined to consist not of perfection or of being better than someone else but of improving on one's own performance. Everyone can attain this goal. Competition is deemphasized, and in fact one of the experiences that the children are taught to enjoy is the accomplishment of being able to help a peer learn something new or devise a good plan for a project. Group esprit and peer relations are thus added to the success experiences.

Programming Attitudes

Many of the cognitive-behavioral techniques used in the group are based on reality therapy and rational emotive therapy concepts. Throughout the group, irrational beliefs are exposed, and more rational attitudes are planted through such techniques as imbedding the message in a question; examples are, "Did you know that _____?" or "How do you explain the fact that _____?" Another technique is abruptly confusing with a pattern disruption and then providing an apparent answer that carries a suggestion as to attitude; for example, "Who can name an electric drug? [blank but curious stares] Give up? I'll tell you. It's television! Television can get you addicted and snow you under like a drug so that all of the good ideas that you have in your mind get kind of drunk. Then the good, sensible thoughts that you all have inside your head somewhere and that you can pull out if you just take time enough to think about them, don't have a chance, while you're watching television. So all you have to do is turn off the television and turn on your brain to find out what you can really do." Other metaphors used include fables such as the boy who cried "wolf."

Analogies are often used: "Some kids learn to swim easily; you just throw them in the water as babies, and they paddle off. They're lucky. Others have to take lessons to swim and may not learn until they're fifteen years old. In the same way, some kids easily learn to sit still, pay attention, control their temper, and plan before they act. Others have to take lessons to learn those things, and it takes them longer to learn. You have to work harder at learning to concentrate and control yourself, and we're giving you special lessons so you can learn, just like the people who need swimming lessons to learn to swim."

Resource Utilization

A study of the differences between achieving and nonachieving children indicated that those who achieve well in school are those who have learned to make use of adults as resources while carrying out many tasks on their own. Nonachievers either continually depend on adults for constant direction or continue to fumble on their own when they should ask for help. The structure of the group teaches appropriate use of adults as resource persons. Children have tasks that they are expected to carry out on their own, on which they are encouraged to ask for help when they become temporarily stumped.

The best example is in picking the project for the coming week; the children have the option of picking their own project or asking for ideas from their parents. Sometimes they are able to ask for ideas from other children in the group or parents other than their own. Also, during the Socratic discussion they are encouraged, when stumped, to ask for some ideas from the parents. The comment is often made that "parents can be good consultants." The parents are taught to take a consultative attitude in contrast to the over-directiveness or rejection that some of them manifest at first visit. They are also taught to see themselves as resources of the children, resources that should be preserved for the most essential matters and not wasted on trivial or unimportant concerns. In this indirect manner the parent's self-esteem is bolstered. Their attitudes and self-concepts are reoriented through some of the same neurolinguistic and hypnotic techniques as with the children. At the same time, they are taught some increased competencies to increase the reality basis for their improved self-esteem as parents.

Feedback

The valuing of both positive and negative feedback contributes to an improved ability to use adults as resources. Many of the children have become deaf to negative feedback because of overkill and overexposure. At the same time, they became suspicious and unaccepting of any positive feedback because of their negative self-image and feelings of unworthiness. Explanations are frequently made of the importance of both positive and negative feedback, and the children are gradually taught to value such feedback rather than feel burdened by it. This allows the parents' natural feedback to be heard by the child.

Modifying the Modifier and Modifee

The focus on feedback is through star charts about the child's performance for that day. (A star chart is a calendar-like matrix with the rows being different accomplishments and the columns different days. Successes are recorded as stars in the appropriate cells.) The public display of the child's stars not only is a further success experience for the child and allows the family to see the child as competent, but it also teaches the family simple behavior modification techniques. Most of the families spontaneously begin using star charts on their own at home after seeing them used effectively in the group. However, the applications of behavior modification are not confined to the star chart. Both parents and children are positively reinforced throughout the group for constructive attitudes, statements, actions, and changes.

Group Techniques

Although this group is far from the usual concept of group therapy, many traditional group therapy techniques are retained, such as going around the room, generalizing, asking the opinion of others about a particular person's problem, facilitation of communication through humor, lowering of anxiety level, and defining of ground rules. The more traditional group techniques find the most appropriate application in the parents' group but are also used in the combined sessions of parents and children.

Sensory Integration and Body Image

Sensory integration activities such as those advocated by Jean Ayres form the core of the separate children's group, though they are modified somewhat to dovetail into the emphasis of the rest of the session.[1] They are used not only for their own value but also as a medium for other therapeutic efforts. Many of the children who come to the group have problems with body image and basic self-handling skills. They consider most of the activities fun even though it is carefully explained to them that these have a purpose and the primary purpose is not to have fun. By going through the activities in a group setting, the children not only improve their coordination, comfort with their body image, and sense of bodily competence, but also improve their social skills in a manner that seems fitted to carry over to the playground and athletic field.

Origin of Structure

The present highly structured, stylized therapeutic format has evolved over eight years, with gradual shaping, mutations, and acquisition of techniques from many sources. When group treatment for behavior and learning problems was first tried, we considered it a kind of experiment. We fully expected problems, knowing that such children were much more difficult to handle in a group than individually. At first we were not disappointed in our expectation of problems. There were times in the beginning when an hour seemed an ordeal, with youngsters flitting in and out of the group room and continually disrupting. At this stage we were attempting traditional unstructured discussion type group therapy with parents and children together.

The first adaptive mutation was having a separate parents' group in the middle of the session. The parents were able to make use of the more orthodox group techniques that we favored at that time, and for a while the parents' group became the most valued and emphasized aspect of the group. At one point it expanded to fill up most of the time, with a very thin slice of window dressing at the beginning and end with the children in order to justify the parents' coming. The separate children's group was essentially a babysitting operation, except for occasional inspiration, such as making a videotape skit to show the parents when they reconvened.

The mutation of second importance was to structure the children's group around sensory integration activities. Within two weeks of introducing sensory integration, the complexion and atmosphere of the group changed dramatically. The children became much calmer and organized. The rest of the clinic, which had previously complained about the disruptiveness and noise from the group, ceased its complaints, and the tentative plans to recruit additional staff to help manage the children's behavior on the mornings of "hyperkinetic group" were dropped.

Other mutations of importance included the reporting of each group to the other, the introduction of assignments or projects, and the systematizing of star charts. The borrowings from Silver and Hagin's program, from neuro-linguistics, and from other sources were gradually added as they came to our awareness.[2] The development of a cognitive-behavioral core philosophy was gradual and present to some degree from the beginning.

Interprofessional Logistics

This group treatment is based on an interprofessional approach and cannot be undertaken single-handedly. Successful execution requires a minimum of three staff. Of these, two should remain with the children's group during the split group phase to provide sufficient structure and allow for the possible need to take children off to the side to settle down or possibly even to restrain one. Three staff for the children's group are even better; with the parent's group leader, this would make a total of four staff.

At least one of the staff needs to be an experienced mental health professional with some knowledge of individual and group dynamics, various psychotherapeutic approaches, family therapy, and behavioral principles. At least one of the staff should be a physician who can provide information and advice about medication effects, rationale, type, and dosage, and the neurophysiological basis of some children's disorders. At least one of the staff needs to be familiar with sensorimotor activities; an occupational therapist is the most likely candidate for this role, though other professional disciplines might provide appropriate background for leading and supervising the children's activity group. Viable interprofessional combinations might thus include a psychiatrist, an occupational therapist, and a nurse or educator; a pediatrician, a psychologist, and an occupational therapist; a psychologist, a family practitioner, and an adaptive physical educator; and a pediatrician, an experienced psychiatric social worker, and an occupational therapist.

Notes

1. A. Jean Ayers, *Sensory Integration and Learning Disorders* (Los Angeles: Western Psychological Services, 1973).

2. A.A. Silver and R.A. Hagin, *Search and Teach* (New York: Walker Education Publishing Company, 1976).

2
First Parent-Child Segment: Staging, Warm-up, and Report

T he beginning segment of the group, though short, is important in establishing the atmosphere and expectations for the remainder of the session. It has four subsections: introductions, optional memory exercises, recitation and reporting of assignments from the previous session, and emphasis on planning.

Introductions

Among the basic principles taught parents are to start at a level where the child is capable of achieving, keep things simple, and take one step at a time. Accordingly we focus first on a simple social skill that many of the children have not bothered to learn but is within their reach: introducing themselves and their parents. As with each subsection, the children are asked what comes next and given a chance to recite; then the veteran group members are asked to show the newcomers how it is done:

Dr. A.: We have a new kid here today. Who can tell him the first thing we have to do?

Tom: Say our name and point to our mother and father.

Dr. A: That's right. Who wants to begin? Do you want to start it, Dick? [Dick happens to be next to the new child. By starting with him and going in the opposite direction, the new child can be the last one up, thereby having the advantage of seeing how the others do the introductions. With this example and the peer pressure and support that has developed by that time, the newcomer is usually able to succeed the first time with the introduction.]

Dick: I'm Dick Jones, and this is my mother (*pointing to her*), and this is my father (*pointing*).

Dr. A.:   (*looking at the next family*) You're next.

Harriet: I'm Harriet Smith, and this is my mother Jane (*pointing*).

Tom: I'm Tom Miller and this is my father and this is my grandmother.

By the time the introductions get around to the newcomer, the child is usually able to make the introduction. Those who hesitate or seem to have trouble are told again simply that they need to say their name and point to their mother and father. If they seem to flounder, they are first told to say their name and then told to point to their mother and father. This demonstrates for the parents the principle of breaking down an overwhelming task into smaller pieces at which the child can succeed. If a child mumbles, the other youngsters are asked if they can hear and are encouraged to ask for louder repetition. If a child cannot respond at all to an adult request, the veteran youngsters in the group are encouraged to ask for the name and even to go over to the silent child for a more intimate request if necessary. Sometimes one of the other children will repeat the name louder for a child who has trouble saying it loud enough. As a last resort, children who are not able to say their name at all are asked if they want their mother or father to say it for them this first time. We have never had a child refuse to nod at this point. They are thus given their first experience of using their parents as a resource person in the group, and the parents are given a taste of being able to help their child. By the second session, all children are able to say their own name.

Optional Memory Exercise

If the group has started on time and seems to be moving along briskly enough so that time will not be a problem, it is desirable to ask the veterans to describe to the newcomer how the group works. The veterans thus have a chance to practice auditory memory and sequencing and experience success in front of the group. Those not speaking at the moment practice careful listening, as well as auditory memory and sequencing, knowing that they will be asked to fill in any parts that the first recitor misses, forgets, or gives in the wrong order. Although a useful technique, this is merely a stronger version of things that are done throughout the group on a more casual basis and can be deleted if time is pressing.

Recitation and Reporting

The next segment, like the others, is introduced by a question:

Dr. E.: Who can tell what comes next?

Dick: We report on our assignments [or projects or homework].

Dr. E.:   And what are the three things you report, Joe?

Joe: Our plan and our goal and how well we did.

Dr. E.:   That's right. Did Joe say them in the right order? [Dick's hand up.] Dick?

Dick: The goal comes first.

Joe: Oh, yeah.

Dr. E.:   Right. First you say your goal, which is what you were going to do, then your plan, which is how you remembered to do it, and then how well you did. Who wants to go first?

Several children may put their hands up, eager to report first. The group leader should take careful note of the order in which the hands went up and take the reports in that order. If several hands are simultaneous, the occasion can be used as a means of teaching the social skill of deciding on turns. A coin flip might be utilized or alphabetical order, with the one who was second getting to go first at the next session or perhaps the one who was second on reporting gets to go first on picking the new assignment at the end of the group. If no one raises a hand, a successful approach has been the following:

Dr. E.:   That's right, Dick. Do you want to go first? [Dick nods.]

Dick: I remembered to do it five days out of seven.

Dr. E.:   First you report your goal, then your plan, and then how well you succeeded.

Dick: My goal was to feed the dog every day without being told. My plan was that when I ate my snack after I came home from school, I would remember that the dog likes to eat, too. I remembered five days out of seven.

Dick's mother: He did it every school day, but on the weekend he didn't have a snack after school, and he forgot those days.

Dr. A.:   So there was a flaw in your plan. Can you think what you can do on a weekend to remember?

Dick: I could use breakfast for the reminder.

Dr. A.:   That's a good idea. You could use your after-school snack during the week and your breakfast on Saturday and Sunday to remind you. But anyhow, five out of seven is good. That's about a .700 batting average, which is terrific even for a big league player.

Success is redefined as anything better than what the child had been doing previously. The analogy to a batting average is a concrete reminder that success does not require perfection. On the occasions that a child does have a totally successful week he or she is given a round of applause in special recognition. On the rare occasions when the child is not able to report a success, the report is accepted in a matter-of-fact manner, but no excuses are accepted:

Harry: I was only able to do it once because my alarm clock was broken . . .

Dr. A.: You don't need to give excuses for why you didn't do it. We're not interested in excuses. We just want to know how many times you did it. You say that you did it once?

Harry: Yes, once.

Dr. A.: Is that more than you did it before?

Harry: Yes, I didn't do it all the week before.

Dr. E.: Well, then that's one more time, 100 percent improvement over what you did before. Very good; keep it up.

Although the child's excuse is not accepted—excuses would sabotage the whole thrust of the group by focusing on perfection of excuses rather than on improvement of behavior—Dr. A. will not disregard the broken alarm clock entirely. He may take it up with Harry's parent in the separate parents' group or at the end of the group may help Harry devise a plan that does not depend on an alarm clock.

The youngster's report is always checked at least nonverbally with the parents. No child takes offense at this, partly because no child is tempted to lie, knowing that the parent, who is present, will be checked with about the report. We are not interested in training children to lie with poise by refusing to check with their parents in a facade of trust. We openly check with the parents in order to provide the children with feedback as to whether their self-perception was accurate. Often before the group convenes, the child and parent discuss the intended report and arrive at a consensus as to what happened. On the rare occasions that the child's report is not corroborated by the parents, we take whatever time is needed to explore the source of misunderstanding. This is done in a spirit of discovery of miscommunicaton and comparison of different perceptions of the truth. No child has responded negatively to this, and it has usually resulted in improved understanding between parent and child. It also demonstrates to all the families that problems can be faced squarely and resolved without the need to assign blame or gloss over problems. Here is an actual transcript; the child's goal had been to avoid fights:

Dr. A.: And how did you do this week?

Kurt E: Great. I didn't get into any fights.

Dr. A.: (*surprised*) Oh, good. Let's check with your mother.

Mrs. E.: No fights, Kurt? That's not right. Meaning you didn't fight at all?

Kurt: One fight, maybe.

Dr. A.: One fight. Is that about right? [Kurt nods.]

Mrs. E.: Well, Kurt, it seemed to me that you did improve, but there was more than one fight. I couldn't really count them.

Kurt: That's a joke!

Dr. A.: (*to group*) How do you think this can be? Over the same two-week period Kurt and his mother say he got into fights a different number of times. It looks like they have a disagreement. Who can help me with this? Craig? How can that be? Can you think of reasons why two people would look at the same thing and say two different things? [Craig shakes his head.]

Kurt: How is she supposed to keep track if she's working?

Dr. A.: You mean she's not around to see? OK; let's check with some of the others. What would be the reason one person would say, "I saw five fights" and the other would say, "I saw one fight"?

Andy: The number of fights. They're sort of fighting right now—arguing.

Dr. A.:   That's very good. Did everybody catch that? They might disagree on what a fight is. Someone might think it's a fight, and the other might think it's just arguing. Let's check and see if that's the explanation.

Mrs. E..:   One thing I can think of, too. Did this mean fighting with other children or fighting with Tom [Kurt's brother], too?

Kurt: It meant fighting with other children.

Dr. A.:   With other kids. Oh, I see.

Mrs. E.:   With other kids? Well, if that's it, then, yes, that's right, Kurt, you really did improve. Maybe you only got into one fight with other kids.

Dr. A.:   You all had a chance to learn something here: that when you think someone is lying because they don't say the same thing you are saying, even if you know you're right, sometimes it may be that words people use don't have the same meanings. For the word *fight*, Kurt meant only fighting with somebody outside the family, but his mother understood fighting with anybody, including brother. We had a chance to find out here that both were right about the number. Also, both saw that Kurt had improved in fighting less.

At the end of the reports, newcomers are told apologetically that we are sorry that they do not have anything to report through no fault of their own, since they were not there the previous time and therefore were not able to pick a project; however, they will have an opportunity to pick a project at the end of this group that they can report on the next time. Having a project to work on is thus presented as a privilege and adventure, and 95 percent of the children accept it as such.

Planning

The final section of the first parent-child segment involves asking the children what comes next. This is a special asking because the moment is loaded with excitement in anticipation of the activities, which most of the children enjoy. This moment of anticipation, excitement, and receptiveness is utilized to get across one of the central thrusts of the group: to think before you act, summarized in one important word, *plan:*

Dr. A.:	All right, what comes next?
Harriet:	The parents go to another room, and the kids go to the gym.
Dr. A.:	That's right, but what do you kids have to do before you go to gym?
Harriet.:	We have to find out what we're going to do.
Dr. A.:	And how do you find out what you're going to do?
Tom:	By asking.
Dick:	And by listening.
Dr. A.:	Very good. I'm glad you remembered the importance of listening. It doesn't do much good to ask if you don't bother listening to the answer, does it? The only way you can know what you're supposed to do is by listening. But what other important step comes between listening to the directions and going to the activities?
Harry:	Voting.
Dr. A.:	Well, that's right. Sometimes Mrs. S. gives you a choice of several activities, and you get a chance to vote so that you don't have to fight with each other about which ones you'll choose. But there is still another very important thing that you need to do between listening to the directions and understanding them and actually doing things. [The children look a bit puzzled.] It's a very important four-letter word that you hear every week. It begins with a *P*. It's a four-letter word, but it's not a dirty word. (*laughter from the parents*), and it's OK for you to say it. Does anybody know? You use it in your projects. You have a goal and you have a . . .
Several children at once:	Plan!
Dr. A.:	That's right. Planning is the most important thing you learn here. If you don't plan something, you can't be sure you are going to do it right. When you plan, you think it

out in your head how you're going to do it, and then you're sure you are going to do it right. Planning keeps you out of trouble and makes things more fun, because then you can do them right. OK. You kids stay here with Mrs. S. and one of the student doctors to plan your activities, while the parents come with me to the other room.

3
The Children's Hour

Katherine Sheridan
L. Eugene Arnold

T he meat of the sandwich is a separate forty to fifty minute children's group running simultaneously with the parents' group. It is highly structured. Sensory integration activities occupy most of the time, with an important planning session at the beginning. During the planning session, the children have an incentive to practice listening and group cooperation. Since most of them enjoy the activities and look forward to them, they are motivated by the fact that the activities will begin only after they complete the planning. Here is a transcript of a planning session, which ordinarily takes about five to ten minutes.

Mrs. S.: Let's all sit together in a circle on the floor. This will make it easier for everyone to hear. [Jack wants to remain in a chair away from the group.] I know the chair is comfortable, but I'd like you to be a part of the group. [Jack joins the circle.]

We have two new children in the group today. I think it would be helpful if we begin by sharing our star charts with them. Do I have a volunteer? [Dora raises her hand.] Dora?

Dora: This is for feedback. It lets you know the things you are doing right and the things you need to do better.

Mrs. S.: Why is it important to know that?

Dora: That way we can keep doing the good things and change the bad things. You can earn stars for . . . [reads the items on the chart], and if you do them halfway, you earn checkmarks.

Mrs. S.: That was very well organized, Dora. You remembered everything. Are there any questions? [There are none.]

Mrs. S.: (*to newcomers*) We need to plan together what we're going to do in the gym. How about some kind of relay races? You can decide what type of races you want. Now that gives you a choice of scooter boards, running, crawling, jumping, hopping, skipping, and walking.

Dora: Scooter boards!

Mrs. S.: I have one suggestion for scooter boards. Are there any other suggestions?

Ernie: I know, the ones where we have a tunnel, jump rope, and scooter boards.

Mrs. S.: You mean an obstacle course?

Group: Yeah! Let's do that.

Mrs. S.: If there aren't any more suggestions, let's take a vote. All those for scooter board races raise your hand. [One raises hand and looks embarrassed for being the only one.] All those for an obstacle course raise your hand. [Eight raise hands.] The obstacle course wins. Now you need to decide how you are going to set up the obstacle course. Do I have a volunteer to write the ideas on the chalkboard?

[Many raise their hands. Jack, a newcomer, is chosen because it would give him a job while the veterans do the bulk of the planning. As it turns out, Jack assumes a strong leadership role.]

Jack: I don't know what you have in the gym to use. [All the children begin telling.]

Mrs. S.: One at a time, please. Eddie, you have the floor.

Eddie: We have jump ropes, mats, a volleyball net, inner tubes, scooter boards, and balls.

Jack: We could . . . [He begins making an involved diagram of an obstacle course on the chalkboard. All the children have turned and are listening intently to his plan.]

Mrs. S.: Jack has presented a suggestion for an obstacle course. What does the group think? [The group shows its approval.] Are there any changes you would make? [All shake their heads.] OK; one last decision before we go to the gym: are we going to have only one obstacle course or two exactly the same so that you can race?

Jack: We can have one and take turns.

Jim: There might not be enough time for everyone to get a chance.

Mrs. S.: If we have one, everyone can watch each other, but everyone must wait quietly for their turn. If we have two courses, everyone will have a chance for sure. Let's take a vote. [The group unanimously decides on two courses.] Everyone planned very well together today. Let's go downstairs [to the gym]. [Everyone lines up at the door and leaves together.]

Setting, Space, and Organization

For many of the activities, a gymnasium is ideal, and since one is available, we make use of it. A large, uncluttered room would usually do as well, since the amount of space in a gym is not necessary, and the basketball hoops are used only rarely. A few of the activities are not suitable for a gym. Some may require a room with some tables (in which case the children might stay awhile in the large group room that the combined group is held in) or may require a kitchen, in which case we use the occupational therapy facilities.

Most of the activities have more than one purpose or value and are probably beneficial to all children in some way. However, the person directing the children's group should be aware of the special needs of the children who are attending and try to design activities especially suitable for them. For example, if most of the children have fine-motor coordination problems, pegboards or marble boards would be good to include. If many of the children seem rather clumsy in keeping their balance, kinesthetic and vestibular activities should be emphasized. At all times, emphasize cooperation with the rest of the group and improving one's own performance rather than competing with others.

Equipment

There is an overwhelming variety and amount of equipment that could benefit the children's group, but most facilities are short of storage space and equipment budget. Our solution has been to be creative with the equipment and supplies readily available, purchasing only a few essentials. Four scooter boards (12 inch × 12 inch × 1 inch boards, each with four 2 inch ball-bearing wheels) and a 15 foot diameter multicolored nylon parachute have been especially valuable. Other useful equipment and supplies include floor mats, sturdy 1 inch diameter long ropes, balls of varying sizes and weights, parking cones, inflated car inner tubes, ladders, chairs, blankets, colored inch cubes with design cards, pegboards, masking tape, rolls of brown wrapping paper, poster and water paints, crayons, styrofoam "peanuts," textured cloth and paper, and clay. Each of these can be used in many ways, limited only by creativity. Special education and recreation suppliers are good resources for equipment and supplies, but many times supplies can be made.

Activity Precautions

Sensory integrative therapy is selecting, controlling, and providing sensory input that will elicit adaptive motor responses. The sensory integration activities we use frequently stimulate the vestibular, proprioceptive, kinesthetic, and tactile systems and may be either excitatory or inhibitory. Children are usually good judges of how activities affect their brain mechanism. Overstimulation can be disorganizing and threatening to the children. No activity should be forced on a child, particularly activities involving vestibular and tactile stimulation. Any activity that causes flushing or blanching of the face, nausea, or unusual perspiring or yawning should be stopped.

Care must be taken to prevent sensory overload, which manifests as overexcitement beyond a half-hour following the treatment session, a destructive approach to the environment, or total withdrawal from the environment. If a child becomes overstimulated, inhibitory and relaxing activities may be introduced, which include slow rhythmical spinning, rocking or stroking, neutral warmth, and deep pressure to the body.

Although occurring infrequently, sensory overinhibition of the brain stem through inhibitory vestibular input could result in stupor and cyanosis from depression of vital functions. Excitatory light touch to the feet and face will help normalize the neurological responses.

Activity Options

Each of the activities presented here can meet a variety of training needs: learning to listen and follow instructions, cooperating with a group, learning social and communication skills, participating in self-expression activities, channeling energies, developing gross- and fine-motor skills, and receiving sensory integrative treatment. The expertise of the therapist in evaluation and treatment of sensory integrative dysfunction will determine how much emphasis is placed on sensory integration.

Sensory integration occurs at a subcortical level in the brain. The children's group therapist should refrain from bringing to the child's consciousness the adaptive response being sought. For example, children with a poorly integrated tonic labyrinthine reflex will drag their legs while riding prone on the scooter board; linear acceleration (for example, pushing off from the wall or riding down a ramp) elicits the adaptive response of automatically assuming a pivot prone (extensor) pattern. If children are merely asked to keep their legs off the ground when riding the scooter board, they will be using their cortex to think consciously about keeping their legs up instead of experiencing the movement patterns. Because chances of integration are lessened when the child consciously focuses on the desired responses, activities are more effective if made into games.

The following is an outline of problem areas commonly treated. Descriptions of suggested activities are included for each area.

Postural Insecurity

Activities for treating postural insecurity, which includes poor integration of the tonic labyrinthine reflex (TLR) and poor equilibrium reactions, should begin low to the ground and keep to the basics, such as rolling, crawling, creeping, and riding scooter boards. As skills improve, work up to activities that take a higher level of neuronal response. This includes walking on balance beams, inner tubes, or vestibular boards.

Activities to Integrate the Tonic Labyrinthine Reflex

1. Playing airplane on the scooter boards, the children spin themselves first in one direction and then the other to facilitate the extensor prone position and provide vestibular stimulation. This can be incorporated into relay races or obstacle courses (*vestibular activity*).
2. Pushing off the wall with both hands or feet while lying prone on the scooter board not only offers proprioceptive and bilateral integrative input but can assist in integration of the TLR from the linear acceleration. Have the child try to push hard enough to reach a certain point. Increase the distance as the skill improves (*proprioception, vestibular perception, and bilateral integration*).
3. The child lying prone on the scooter board may be pulled in an arc around the therapist by both therapist's and child's holding on to an inner tube or rope. The therapist is the pivot in this activity and will also receive vestibular stimulation. This stimulation can be a disadvantage to therapists who cannot tolerate spinning. In groups, the children can work with each other (*vestibular, co-contraction, and bilateral integration*).
4. When playing boat on the scooter boards, the children pull themselves along a rope tied so that it is taut about 18 inches from the floor. This activity can be performed in either a supine or a prone position. When

supine, the adaptive response will be a flexor pattern (*co-contraction, kinesthesia*).

5. Hoop toss: Hold a hoop about 12–18 inches away from and above the head of the child lying prone on a scooter board. With both hands at once, the child picks up a rubber ring or beanbag and tosses it through the hoop. The higher the children reach, the more likely they will begin assuming the desired prone extensor position in tossing the ring (*bilateral integration*).

Activities to Promote Righting and Equilibrium Reactions

1. Inner tube roll: Tape or tie five tire inner tubes together. The child lies inside with head out and rolls in the tubes. To encourage righting ask the child to look for a certain point on the wall toward which he or she is rolling. This activity also provides vestibular and touch-pressure stimulation (*righting response*).
2. Rolling up in blankets, in the parachute, or on mats can be included in obstacle courses or relay races (*righting*).
3. King of the tube: Kneeling on inner tubes, the children try to push each other off balance while maintaining their own balance. As the child gains skill, this activity could be tried standing up (*equilibrium*).
4. Play catch or four square while kneeling or standing on inner tubes. Purposely toss the ball high, low, or to the side to add challenge (*equilibrium*).
5. Walking and bouncing on the inner tubes (*equilibrium, bilateral integrating when bouncing*).
6. Toeing the line: Tape a long 1 to 1½ inch diameter rope to the floor. Walk on it as a tightrope (*equilibrium*).
7. Musical chairs using objects of varying heights to sit on. The children should refrain from using their hands to find the seat.
8. Sidewalk serpent: The child holds on to a rope while sitting or kneeling on a scooter board. The therapist then pulls the child in a variety of directions and speeds (*co-contraction, equilibrium, proprioception*).
9. Twister is a commercially available game that requires the child to maintain balance in a variety of unusual positions. The game consists of a large sheet of plastic with colored dots and a spinner board that indicates on which colored dot the child is to place the designated hand or foot (*equilibrium, right-left discrimination, praxis*).
10. Balance beam: Have the child focus on a stationary object so that balancing is a function of tactile and proprioceptive feedback instead of visual (*equilibrium*).

Other Activities to Promote Postural Security

1. Animal walks: These can be used in obstacle courses or relay races:

    Duck walk: Walk while squatting low to the floor.

    Crab walk: Walk on all fours but with the torso supine; keep the buttocks off the floor (*proprioception*).

    Elephant walk: The hands are clasped with the arms outstretched to form a trunk. While walking bent over, the trunk is swung from side to side (*crossing the midline*).

    Camel walk: Walk on all fours but with the extremities extended.

    Bunny hop: With both feet together, arms are held out in front like rabbit forepaws (*bilateral integration*).

    Kangaroo hop: Jump or hop with an object held between the knees (*bilateral integration*).

2. Clap out patterns or rhythms demonstrated by the leader (*bilateral integration; if eyes are closed, this will also help auditory sequencing*).
3. Use the scooterboard as a surfboard, paddling across the floor with both arms simultaneously (*bilateral integration*).
4. Do-si-do: Standing in a circle, everyone faces the same direction (clockwise or counterclockwise) with one shoulder to the center. A large ball is passed around the circle in a pattern of over one head and then under and between the next person's legs.
5. Water walk: The parachute is held open by the outer edge at waist level. Everyone then whips arms up and down to create "waves" in the parachute. One to three children are then allowed in the center to walk or roll on the "waves." Caution: Do not allow the children on the outside of the parachute to pull the chute out from under the walkers' feet. This activity provides both proprioception and light touch tactile stimulation. If it becomes overstimulating, move on to a different activity or follow with calming techniques.
6. Merry-go-run: Each person maintains a hold on the outer edge of the parachute. Starting at the floor level, on the count of three everyone raises the chute. As the chute peaks, everyone runs around the perimeter back to the original spot before the chute falls.

Tactile Defensiveness

Tactile defensiveness is associated with disturbance in the protopathic or protective tactile system. It is manifested by touch avoidance, hyperactivity, distractibility, poor tactile discrimination, and poor behavior during tactile activities. Defensive children are often unaware of the distress they feel during tactile activities, but some of their comments can provide clues: "It tickles," "It hurts," "Can I get a drink?" "When can we stop?" or "I hate this game."

Because of the intense responses, tactile stimulation is usually offered at the beginning of a session so that the response can be accurately monitored before the child goes home. Defensive responses can be diminished by incorporating tactile stimulation into proprioceptive and vestibular activities, by having the child self-impose the stimulation, or by focusing on the games instead of the stimulation provided. Let the children and their behavior judge when to terminate specific tactile activities.

Methods and Activities to Normalize the Protective Tactile System

1. Soft or subliminal sell: Tactile stimulation may be made an inherent part of many activities simply by covering scooter boards with shag carpet, playing hopscotch on carpet samples, covering floor mats with blankets, lining barrels or tunnels with textured fabrics, or playing catch with textured fabric balls. By ensuring that the tactile experiences are not a point of focus, you can help the defensive child more easily tolerate such experiences.
2. Do-it-yourself: Tactile stimulation is less threatening when self-imposed. Children can brush their body parts with paint brushes or textured fabrics such as terrycloth, fleece, corduroy, or velvet. They can rub on body lotion or baby powder. A variation is to have the children pretend they are swimming, then hop out of the pool, and dry off their whole body with their fabric. This fantasy can be played on a carpeted floor; the floor becomes their towel.
3. Erasure: Mark various spots on the children's arms and legs with chalk or adhesive coding dots. Have them erase the marks with textured fabric.
4. Back rubs or back scratching.
5. Upright rolling along a wall can provide touch pressure, particularly to the shoulders and back. This is easily incorporated into an obstacle course.
6. People sandwich: A group of children lie prone, flat on a mat. Place another mat on top of the group, making sure the heads are free. Another group of children roll on top of the sandwich, avoiding the heads. Do not force participation. This activity provides vestibular stimulation for the rollers and calming deep pressure for those in the sandwich.
7. The feely bag, as described under tactile discrimination, provides a good deal of desensitizing, normalizing stimulation to the protective system.

8. Parachute games, in which the body contacts the chute by walking or rolling in and under it, provide light touch.
9. Finger painting.

Apraxia

A good body scheme is essential for development of praxis. If the brain does not perceive the body as a motor instrument, it cannot accurately plan and execute coordinated nonhabitual motor tasks. Activities to counteract apraxia (poor motor planning) should be unfamiliar and ever changing to promote sensory integration rather than mere splinter skill development. Kinesthetic, vestibular, and tactile awareness are important components of body scheme development. Activities to normalize the vestibular system have already been identified; the focus here will be on tactile and kinesthetic functions.

Activities to Develop Tactile Discrimination. The epicritic or discriminative tactile system is most closely associated with praxis. For tactilely defensive children, see suggestions in the previous section to normalize the protopathic or protective tactile system before moving on to the higher discriminative level.

1. Matching textures: Glue different textured papers and fabric to 3 x 5 cards. Use several fabrics of each texture with different appearance. Have the children sort the cards according to texture.
2. Tactile description: Categorize different objects by their weight, shape, and texture by handling them. Examples are heavy (bolt, paperweight) versus light (screw, paper clip), soft (cotton, velvet) versus rough (sandpaper), and round (circle, ball, oval) versus square (cube, pyramid).
3. Finger painting or foot painting: Add to the paint sand, cornmeal, starch, or similar substance to change the texture.
4. Feely bag: Conceal common objects in a fabric bag (a pillow case will do; burlap will provide extra stimulation) that has been filled with Styrofoam peanuts. Each child in turn places a hand in the bag, identifies one object, and pulls it out to see if he or she is right (*includes normalization of protopathic touch because of nondiscriminatory contact with the bag, peanuts, and other objects*).
   A variation is for each child in turn to pull out and show an object from the feely bag. He or she then replaces the object, shakes the bag to hide it, and gives the bag to the next child to retrieve the object by touch.
   A second variation is to hide objects in a sandbox.
5. Bread pretzels: This activity is generally enjoyed by all of the children because they have an opportunity to cook and can eat the products of

their labor. Encourage the children to make a variety of shapes with the dough (*includes protopathic touch normalization*). Here is the recipe:

1. Preheat oven to 425°.
2. Mix 1 package dry yeast with 1 1/2 cups warm water. Add 1 tablespoon sugar, 1 teaspoon salt, and 4 cups of flour.
3. Mix the dough with hands and knead well. The dough is ready when it no longer sticks to fingers and is smooth and elastic. Dough can be kneaded endlessly without hurting it.
4. Shape pretzels and place on ungreased cookie sheet.
5. Glaze with beaten egg, and sprinkle with coarse salt.
6. Bake for 12 to 15 minutes or until pretzels are light brown.

Activities to Develop Kinesthesia

1. Isometric exercises are helpful for kinesthesia because of proprioceptive input. Make the exercises fun by using imagination. For example, pretend to make a room larger by pushing out the walls and floor.
2. Push-of-war: Place a tape line on the floor. The children, working in pairs, try to cross the line by pushing the partner. They can use different body parts: both hands together, elbows together, hips, feet, or backs. A variation is to try to push a sturdy box over the line against the partner's resistance.
3. Heavy scooting: Do scooter board activities with weighted cuffs around the wrists or ankles.
4. Hot potato: Use a children's-size medicine ball. For a variation, the children, sitting on the floor, pass the medicine ball with different body parts: feet, hands, crook of the elbow.
5. Freeze tag: When tagged, the child must remain in the exact position tagged until unfrozen by another player's touch.
6. Row boat: Children pair up sitting opposite each other, legs apart, feet touching, and holding hands. To row the boat, they rock each other back and forth. If done slowly, this can be calming from the slow, rythmical rocking.

Gross Motor Planning Activities. These activities involve performing several tasks quickly and at once. Most of them also include at least two of the activity types described above (kinesthetic, vestibular, or tactile).

1. Obstacle courses are an excellent way to work on motor planning because they use a series of different activities and experiences. Here is one example of an obstacle course:

Spin five times on the scooter board (*vestibular*).

Push off the wall to reach the mats (8 feet away or adjusted to child's ability) (*proprioception, bilateral integration*).

Pick up five rubber rings along the way (*active motor planning*).

At the mat, throw rings into a box (*visual-motor*).

Roll on the mat to the end of it (*vestibular, tactile*).

Walk on the inner tubes (*equilibrium*).

Crawl through a tunnel made with mats, chairs draped with blankets, or any other convenient equipment (*tactile*).

Hop in and out of a coned circle (*visual-motor, postural security*).

Jump rope to the beginning of the course (*proprioceptive, postural security*).

Sit on the floor when finished.

2. Trick riding: While riding the scooter board, knock over boxes, pick up objects, or weave in and out of cones without touching the cones.
3. Simon says: The child must imitate postures or motions that "Simon says" to do. If Simon does not say, then the child does not imitate (*auditory-visual-motor integration*).
4. Poison: Go through an obstacle course without touching the sides of the tunnel, rungs of a horizontal ladder, or cones that are placed closely together.
5. Snake: Two people hold the end of a jump rope and make it wiggle and ripple along the floor. One at a time, each child jumps back and forth over the rope without landing on it.
6. Hopscotch: As a variation, land on toes for even numbers and heels for odd numbers.
7. Charades (pantomimes): Imitate animals; activities of daily living, such as eating, putting on clothes, or brushing teeth; professions, such as dentist, cashier, or firefighter. The opposite team or whole group guesses what is being imitated.
8. Group knot: The children stand in a circle and mix their hands all together in the center. After a couple of minutes, they are asked to clasp hands with two other people. Without letting go at any time, they are to unscramble themselves. The end result should be a large circle. Sometimes there will be two circles. Because this task is so difficult, the group applauds at the end. The activity, also good for group cooperation, should not be forced.

9. Mirroring: Divide the group into pairs. In each pair, one child is designated leader and the other the mirror. The leader is to explore as many movements as possible, including facial expression. The mirror must follow the leader exactly. After a few minutes, the partners switch roles.

Fine-Motor Planning Activities. These fine-motor activities for eye-hand coordination are often used at the end of a session as a way to calm and channel the stimulation received earlier in the session. Individual table activities also encourage quiet, calm behavior.

1. Matching or duplicating colored block designs or pegboard designs. Or instead of using the blocks, have the children use each other as blocks for a large-scale manipulation of space and form.
2. Weaving potholders or paper.
3. Craft activities that require manipulation of tools. Examples are small wood projects or painting projects.
4. Tracing designs: Pass the design: have the child draw a free-form design and then pass it to the next child to trace.
5. Stringing beads of different shapes and colors, following different patterns.
6. Sorting various small objects into separate small boxes.

A Combination Activity. *Self-portraits:* The leader needs to provide brown wrapping paper (cut in lengths according to each child's height), crayons, and a floor-length mirror. The children lie face up on the paper. Trace around each child (children can help), following the contours of clothing and hair. The children then fill in the outline so that it looks just like themselves. Encourage use of the full-length mirror to determine hair and eye color and where clothing begins and ends.

Hyperactivity or Overstimulation

On occasion, the children arrive at group overstimulated, perhaps by anticipation of holidays. On these days, the therapist needs to incorporate calming activities. These are also good to end sessions. Activity components are slow, rhythmical rocking or stroking, neutral warmth, deep pressure, and decreased environmental stimuli.

Activities That Promote Relaxation

1. Hot dog roll: This activity, enjoyed by most children, has been successfully used by parents at home after seeing it demonstrated in group. The children individually roll up tightly in a cotton blanket with their head

out. Each child is now a hot dog in a bun. The therapist puts on the condiments by slow stroking the child's back with firm, deep pressure along the spinal column. The first hand begins at the nape of the neck. Just as it is about to reach the base of the back, the second hand is placed at the nape of the neck ready to start the second stroke. As the second hand begins, the first is lifted so that the stroking is smooth and continuous. Three minutes is adequate time for this activity; do not overdo it. Watch for overinhibition, such as drowsiness. A variation is to roll a large ball down the person's whole body, using pressure on the ball.

2. Making a tent: Everyone holds on to the outer edge of the parachute. On the count of three, the parachute is lifted above the heads. As it fills with air, it is pulled down and behind everyone's back so that it can be sat on. It is now a tent. For a variation, have the children lean back slightly to find a point of mutual support and then gently sway from side to side in a group rhythm. Be sure to stay in the tent until everyone is quiet.

3. Making a flowerbud or cocoon: One to three people stand on the center of the parachute. The others pull the parachute taut and walk slowly around those in the center until the chute is firmly wrapped to the top of their shoulders. As the direction is reversed and the chute unwrapped, those in the center emerge from the parachute to become flowers or butterflies (*also provides vestibular, proprioceptive, and tactile stimulation*).

4. People spinner: One or two people lie in the center of the parachute. Those on the outside of the chute pull it taut and walk slowly in a circle for a couple of minutes and then reverse directions. This will turn the people in the middle. Be sure everyone is tolerating the vestibular stimulation well. For a variation, have the people in the center sit.

5. Finding your center: Everyone stands in a circle with arms resting. Feet should be approximately a shoulder's width apart. The group is instructed to sway gently from side to side in an over-and-up motion as far as possible without falling or leaning on the next person. Use the following progression for a continuous group sway. Remember to sway slowly.

Sway from side to side with feet firmly planted.

Sway over and up far enough to raise the heel of the opposite foot at the peak of your sway.

Sway raising the opposite foot and standing on the toes of the remaining foot at peak height.

Reverse the order back to the first step.

Close eyes and continue to sway with feet firmly planted.

With eyes still closed, feel the group rhythm and slowly stop together. Each person should end in a centered position (*vestibular stimulation and postural security*).

6. Bear hugs provide firm, deep pressure and happy feelings. Use preventatively, especially when you see a child beginning to get overstimulated.
7. Table games and activities (block designs, pegboard, marble board) can be calming because of the concentration they require. Individual activities may be necessary for these because of children's varying abilities.

Poor Social and Group Skills

Many of the children have been referred to the group for their inability to get along with others. Other chapters describe many opportunities to develop social and group skills. The following activities have been ways for the children to learn and practice these skills.

Activities to Promote Social Skills

1. Name ball: This is particularly useful when there are new members in the group. As the ball is passed from person to person, the children must say their own name first and then the person's name to whom they are passing the ball, for example, "Jack to Ernie," "Ernie to Tom." The staff joins in the circle and sets an example. One variation (*loudspeaker*) is used to practice use of appropriate voice volume. The child speaks in a soft voice when passing the ball to the next child, a medium voice for those a couple of people away, and a playground voice for passing the ball across the circle. In another variation (*Eye Ball*) designed to practice eye contact, the ball is passed without speaking but only when direct eye contact is made with the other person.
2. Quick-change artists: On the count of three, everyone raises the parachute to make a canopy. When it is at the peak, filled with air, the leader calls out the names of two people, who exchange places before the chute falls. Everyone else continues to hold on to the outer edge. As the two exchange places, they shake hands and say "Hi" in the center.
3. Role playing or charades on how to behave in certain situations: Examples are how to use table manners, how to handle a fight, how to behave while shopping with parents, how to make a friend, and how to use the telephone.
4. Barter scavenging: Everyone in the group is given a small object and a pictoral or written checklist of all the items available in the group. The object is to obtain each item for a short period of time so that it can be checked off the list. The only way to obtain an item is to ask politely to exchange objects with another person and then say "thank you." If neces-

sary to keep the group in reasonable control, the leader may decide to have the children take turns.

Activities to Promote Group Cooperation

1. Group collage: Provide a single large sheet of paper, several magazines, scissors, and containers of glue. Do not provide enough supplies to go around; thereby sharing must occur. The group may also decide on a theme. A variation is group painting or drawing.
2. Bread pretzels: The group is expected to share tasks in preparation of the dough, share the dough for kneading and shaping, and work together in clean-up.
3. All parachute games require cooperation to be successful.
4. Group decision making: Usually the children help plan the activities for the day. At this time, they are given guidance on how to offer suggestions to the group, listen to other's ideas, take votes, and determine workable compromises.

The spirit of cooperation that is cultivated in the children's group is further cultivated in the last parent-child segment, when the children and parents are brought back together. In most cases, the cooperativeness, with staff encouragement and structure, spills over into relations with parents as well as with peers.

Note

The reader is referred to these books for further information:

A. Jean Ayers, *Sensory Integration and Learning Disorders* (Los Angeles: Western Psychological Services, 1973).

A. Henderson, L. Lloresn, and E. Gilfoyle, *The Development of Sensory Integrative Theory and Practice* (Dubuque, Iowa: Kendall/Hunt, 1974), esp. pp. 145, 231–235, 240.

Appendix 3A
Equipment Resources

It is not necessary to buy a lot of equipment. Much of the equipment mentioned in this chapter can be scavenged or made by volunteers, staff, or even older children.

Incentive for Learning, Inc.
600 West Van Buren Street
Chicago, Illinois 60607

Motor Education Equipment for Special Populations
Flaghouse, Inc.
18 West 18th Street
New York, New York 10011

Motor Perceptual Equipment, UCS, Inc.
155 State Street
Hackensack, New Jersey 07601

Special Education Materials, Inc.
(an affiliate of G.E. Miller, Inc.)
484 South Broadway
P.O. Box 266
Yonkers, New York 10705

Southpaw Enterprises, Inc.
800 West Third
Dayton, Ohio 45407

4
The Parents' Group

The parents' group runs simultaneously with the children's group, both sandwiched between the combined parent-child sessions. It lasts between forty and fifty minutes.

The parents' group is the least structured part of the whole format. It often resembles traditional group therapy, with ventilation, mutual support, interpretation by group members or the leader, advice from one group member to another, and general sharing of feelings. At other times it tends more in an educational direction, occasionally with question-the-expert, chalk talks, or minilectures by the group leader on a topic of parental concern or misunderstanding.[1]

Behavioral Principles

One of the commonest foci of either chalk talks or less formal educational responses to the parents is behavioral management. Behavioral management principles are explained, including variability of types of reinforcement, reinforcement hierarchies, the advantages of reward over punishment, the most effective use of punishment, the principles of breaking things down into manageable-sized pieces, clear directions, consistency, and setting of priorities.

Dr. A.:   Mrs. T. says she uses ice cream, Mrs. J. said she uses stars on a chart, Mr. U. says he finds that the opportunity to play checkers is very reinforcing to his son, and then some of you have complained about paying the child for doing what he should be doing. Maybe it would be useful to take a look at the hierarchy of reinforcement options that you can use.

At a very elementary level, of course, you have things like tangible reinforcers. These are things like food, drink, warmth, pleasant tactile or vestibular stimulation, sex (of course, for kids we won't include that)—anything that is directly stimulating or meeting a basic physiological need or drive. At the other extreme we would have the feeling of mastery, which is what we would like to see children operate on. They behave well because it makes them feel good; they enjoy being mature; they like the feeling of accomplishment. An example is the toddler who learns to master the toilet and has a feeling of self-control. In between we have a whole spectrum of things.

We have token reinforcers to make a bridge from the more tangible to more abstract psychological reinforcers. Tokens can be things like money or points on a chart that the child earns to get a tangible reinforcer. The next level is social approval, which could include tangible reinforcers such as a pat or a hug, as well as smiles or praise. Some social approval comes very close to the feeling of mastery, which is a kind of self-approval. Social approval includes trust.

One of the things that is important is to help the child progress from the tangible level. Adults at times still operate on the tangible or token level; none of us would continue working over a long period of time if we didn't get our paycheck. We also operate on the level of mastery and self-approval. We need to help the child move from the tangible level to the self-mastery level. The way to do that is to associate them or chain them together. When you give a dish of ice cream at the tangible level, it is important to say "good job" or offer some other less tangible, psychological reinforcer.

After the child values approval or social rewards, then you can begin to change the social reward into something like, "You must feel good that you are able to do a good job on that; you must be proud of yourself." This is a social approval reinforcer couched in terms that will tend to awaken within the child or tune into any flicker of joy in mastery and accomplishment.

Mrs. F.:   I see your point about the tokens and reinforcers, but what can I do about Bobby wanting money for chores I think he should just be doing?

Dr. A.:   The reward doesn't have to be something beyond what you were willing to give in the first place. If you're already doling out fifty cents a week for candy or if you're already taking him to one movie a week, then he needs to earn that. For example, he gets a nickel credit on his allowance each time he carries out the garbage. Take what you would have given him anyway, and set it up in a system where he earns it. This helps him attain self-mastery because he will feel like it is his, and he will know what it means to him. After a while, he may just start doing the chores not only for the money but for your approval. I should mention, too, that if your child is already operating on the social approval level, then you don't have to go back to something tangible. By all means continue with the stage he is at and continue working toward the next level.

Medication

Another important topic is medication. Some of the parents bring their children because they are looking for medicine; some bring them because they are trying to avoid medicine and have heard that we offer other treatments. Some out of each category end up taking medicine, and some of each category do not take medicine. A frank discussion of side effects, actions, and expectations and limitations of medicine helps those who do not wish medicine but whose children should have it to accept it, helps those who want it inappropriately to give it up, and helps those who want it appropriately to use it more wisely and safely.

Parents are cautioned about the following pitfalls in the use of medication:

1. Coming to depend on it to the exclusion of other management techniques.
2. Forgetting to look for psychological explanations for deteriorations in the child's behavior in favor of wanting to have the dosage adjusted.
3. Using the medicine as a means of controlling the child rather than as a means of shoring up the child's self-control and autonomy.
4. Expecting the medicine to make the child perfect even though children without behavior or learning disorders are not perfect.
5. Failing to offer children support in changing their role from bad actor to well-behaved child.
6. Failing to adjust the disciplinary approach to the greater sensitivity of the medicated child.

The Bottomless Pit

The need to recognize, admit, and be comfortable with their own limitations and inability to be perfect parents is another important topic. Many of the children are bottomless pits the parents mistakenly believe they need to fill in order to be good parents.

Mrs. X.: What can you do about the abyss?

Dr. A.: The bottomless pit?

Mrs. X.: Yes. It seems like you just cannot fill it. Don wants more and more, and we seem to do everything for him, but it's just not enough. How can we satisfy him? [Five other parents nod and confirm a similar experience.]

Dr. A.: This is a common problem, not only with behavior-disordered kids but also with other children. You find that they demand and demand. The more you give them, the more they demand. It's kind of like they get hooked or addicted on your giving. They want more and more, and you kind of get drained out. You just don't have any more to give, and they are still demanding, wheedling, and coaxing.

I've noticed that when the kids get really anxious is when they know the parent is drained and can't give any more; then they feel more insecure, and they want more. This leads to a vicious cycle where you feel drained all the time so you don't voluntarily give them anything, and the kid is always demanding so that every time he gets something, it is right after he demanded, so he kind of gets reinforced for demanding. Since you don't have anything left to give voluntarily, the only time he gets anything is when he demands it. He extracts it; he sucks it out of you, and you don't feel like giving voluntarily. This makes a kid more and more demanding and makes you feel less and less like giving.

Rather than try to satisfy, what you have to do is decide ahead of time what it is you can give, where the limits are, and then freely give that before the kid can ask you. Once you've given that, then you have to be firm about not giving anymore, so that he will find out it won't do him any good to demand, wheedle, or coax once you've given what you can. He'll learn to enjoy what he has while he can, and then when you're able to give more, you'll voluntarily give that. He'll learn he doesn't have to keep demanding to get his share. It's hard to give voluntarily when you resent being drained, and it's hard to hold the line against the demanding, wheedling pressure, but that's what's necessary to break up this vicious cycle of child demanding, drained parent withholding, and insecure child demanding more.

Responsibility and Passive Aggression

A recurring question in parents' group is "How do you get kids to _____." The basic problem is the assumption of parental responsibility.

Many parents are relieved when given permission to allow the children to take the consequences of their own failure to act rather than feeling that it is the parents' problem that they are not acting. Parents also need to be attuned to the value of catching the child doing the right thing and reinforcing him or her for it; complete indifference is not the desired attitude. Only the worry, assumption of responsibility, and attempts to coerce the child are counterproductive. The parents' sincere interest in the child is usually helpful. Often another parent is able to get this message across to an overly conscientious parent better than the group leader. Examples of cotherapy by parents in the group can be found in the clinical vignettes in part II.

Witness

Sometimes the parents' group shows flashes of testimony reminiscent of a revival meeting or religious conversion. Here is an example:

Mrs. W.: I used to feel the same way as you do, Mrs. R. I was always fussing with my son, Jerry. It seemed like he was always doing things wrong, and I was always suspecting him and looking for him to do things wrong. Then I noticed that Dr. E. always seemed to be on the kids' side. It wasn't that she was against the parents; she was just seeing things from the kids' viewpoint. Then I got to thinking, "Why shouldn't I be on Jerry's side? I'm his mother, and I should be on his side more than the doctor." So I started looking for ways that I could be on Jerry's side. Now Dr. E. and I are both on Jerry's side, and he's on my side since I'm on his. We still fuss some, but we're not enemies.

What parent could resist that kind of personal witness? The same effectiveness and degree of persuasion could not (and by professional standards perhaps should not) be attained by a professional counselor.

Some Structural Considerations

Although the parents' group is the least structured of the components in this group therapy, even here there is a basic format.

Separation

One of the first items that may require attention is the separation of the parent from the child. This is ordinarily not a problem, but occasionally a child manifests oppositional behavior or merely hostility about being brought to the group the first time by refusing to leave the room where the parent is. Other children, because of repeated failures or immaturity, may cling. Therefore, we prevent problems by having the parents leave the children so that the separation occurs in a passive way for the child. An occasional parent may be reluctant to leave the child, but this is easily handled by expectation and firmness, along with the example of the other parents leaving.

Introductions

A second consideration is to make sure that all of the parents know each other. This is obviously important where a new parent is in the group, but since consistent attendance every week is not required, even some parents who had attended once or twice previously may not have met. Introductions may seem so obvious as not to need mention, but the fact that the children had already introduced themselves and their parents (by pointing), and the fact that the parents' group starts after the group has already been in session for ten or fifteen minutes, easily lead to a mistaken feeling that people already know each other or have already been introduced. Thus it is easy to overlook introductions, which are important in putting the parents at ease at a time when they may feel defensive at the prospect of having to bare their problems in front of others.

Debunking

If the leader senses that many parents in the group are still fearful that mental health professionals blame parents for the problems of their children, it is advisable to make some direct reference early in the group to that myth and make it clear either implicitly or explicitly that this particular mental health professional has seen enough children's problems to know that they are not all the fault of the parents.

Kindling

After introductions, some parents may have an item of business that they wish to bring up, perhaps a problem that has developed the past week or an announcement that things are going well enough that they are planning to reduce their frequency of attendance or even terminate. If no parent has such an issue to bring up, the group leader needs to get things started and help the parents to feel enough at ease to begin sharing. One way to accomplish this is to ask each parent to say a bit about his or her child. This can even be done during introduction.

Another way is to outline some of the possibilities:

This group can be used in any way that you wish. You can use it for com-
miserating, sharing problems—"misery loves company"—reporting of a success, asking for help with a specific problem, developing a behavioral
management plan, trading notes about what seems to work and what doesn't
work, question the expert—and probably find out that the expert doesn't
know much more about it than you do—discussing how to deal with your
child's school, talking about diet or medicine, or even choosing a project for
yourself like the kids do. Projects people have chosen in the past generally fall
into three categories: something to help the child with his or her project, a
separate project to change something about the child's behavior unrelated to
his own project, or a personal project for self-improvement, which you could
share with the child as an example.

If no one picks up on one of the ideas in this explanation of the group's
purpose, the leader can comment on something observed in the first segment
of the group about one of the children: a success that the child had or the fact
that she seemed depressed or disappointed or had not done as well as
previously. Another possibility is to ask the new parent in the group the age
of the child and to comment on which other children represented in the group
are the same age. This usually gets those two or three parents talking to each
other, at least in a *"PTA" fashion*. (PTA is the name of one of the games
described by Eric Berne,[2] in which adults complain, gossip, or brag about
children.)

Limiting Gossip

As a way of fostering interaction, it is acceptable to allow or even promote
five minutes or so of "PTA." This even has some therapeutic value in letting
the parents know their own child is not uniquely disastrous. If this continues
more than ten minutes, the leader should take some definite action to turn the
discussion into a more constructive direction. One way is to focus on the
positive aspects of what has been said, either something good implied about
the child or something good that the parent has done in response to the child.
Another is to clarify the lessons that have been learned. Another is to ask the
other parents in the group to offer suggestions to resolve a problem that one
parent has brought up, perhaps helping that parent formulate a behavioral
management plan. As a last resort, the leader can philosophize about how
growing up is a long, arduous process, with two steps forward and one back,
and how this tries the patience of the parents, and then pose questions as to
how the parents can best assist their children.

This principle does not imply that the parents should be stopped from ventilating their own frustration, disappointments, pressures, anger, or other feelings that result from dealing with their child's problems. Such ventilation can be useful, in contrast to merely gossiping about the children or their escapades or possibly even scapegoating a child. Gossiping and scapegoating need to be limited; ventilation of the parents' own feelings can be not only tolerated, but encouraged.

Quantification and Proportionality of Leader's Participation

Many parents, especially those present for the first time, expect something from the group leader, as well as from the other parents. This is not an unreasonable expectation in view of the fact that most of the parents come seeking information and guidance and are paying a fee for help. Much information and guidance, of course, can come from other parents, but usually something comes up in each group that the leader is the most appropriate person to deal with either by virtue of professional expertise and knowledge or because of the need to have it said by someone in a position of authority.

Generally we have found that the most successful parents' groups have had at least one but not more than two minilectures by the leader. Two examples of minilecture are the earlier description of the reward hierarchy and the bottomless pit discussion. Here is another, which also constitutes an example of reframing. Mrs. X. had been ventilating her frustration about how her son never seems satisfied or grateful. She and his father sacrifice much for him, but he still misbehaves and pesters. This behavior seems all the more ungrateful because a neighbor girl, Ada, behaves well even though neglected by a harsh, unloving mother.

Dr. A.: This is one of the things a lot of people don't understand. You're trying to do everything to be a good parent; you're giving them everything they need in material ways and also by giving your time and energy. You give them the best medical help if they need it and the best psychiatric help if they need it. You spend time with them. You buy things for them and seem to do everything for them, and then they don't seem to appreciate it. They misbehave or throw it back in your face. In a way, maybe you could take it as a compliment, because it seems as if they feel secure enough that they can risk misbehaving. They have confidence in you that you will not abandon them and that you're going to stick with them. If a youngster is really insecure and cannot take any chances with you, then they don't dare disappoint you—as in Ada's case. She always has to be looking out to please her mother, trying to get from her the love and affection that she's not sure she can count on. Then in a sense your children's misbehavior can be looked at as a subtle compliment for the fact that you make them feel secure enough to risk acting that way.

These minilectures need to be presented in such a way as not to quash the parents' inclination to discuss. It is desirable to turn the floor back over to the parents at the end, for example, by saying, "Let's go around and take a security poll. How nasty do your kids feel safe enough to be with you?" or "Perhaps we could go around and have each person share experiences with different types of rewards. Each child is a bit different, and what works with one may not work with another."

Home Base Maneuver

We need to mention a room-hopping peculiarity that has developed in our program out of scheduling necessity but in retrospect we feel may have enough psychodynamic significance that it could be a therapeutic factor. For the split of parents from children to the separate groups, we take the parents to another room, leaving the main group room to the children for planning the activities that they will be carrying out. Usually the children's activities require the gym, so they eventually also vacate the main group room.

The only other room available for the parents' separate group was a classroom of the inpatient school, which was not used during the first class period. The parents' group could use that room until second class, by which time the children generally had vacated the main group room to move to the gym. At that point, the parents moved back to the main group room and continued to discuss whatever topic they were on until the children returned from the gym. This explains the apparent paradox in some of the clinical description chapters that talk about the parents leaving to have their separate group and later having their discussion interrupted by the children returning to the room.

Of more importance, however, is the fact that we have a weekly phenomenon of the parents leaving the children and the children returning to find the parents almost magically back in the same room that they had left the child in. We cannot help but feel that this has some sort of unconscious meaning, perhaps reassurance. Out belief about this is buttressed by the positive atmosphere that prevails on return of the children to find their parents, which is often in contrast to a more negative atmosphere prior to the separate groups. It is also compatible with the comment on follow-up by one mother that the most important part of coming to the group for her family was, "You brought us back together."

We are not sure how much this room hopping may have serendipitously contributed to the efficacy of treatment, but we suggest that if the physical facilities are convenient, it be incorporated into any replication of our program, at least until a study can be designed to tease out its importance.

Notes

1. L.E. Arnold, M. Rowe, and H.A. Tolbert, "Parents' Groups," in *Helping Parents Help Their Children,* ed. L.E. Arnold (New York: Brunner/Mazel, Inc., 1978).

2. E. Berne, *Games People Play* (New York: Ballantine, 1978).

5
The Final Parent-Child Segment

T his last segment of the group, with parents and children back together again, takes thirty to forty-five minutes. It is the most challenging part of the group but also the most fun and the most crucial because it plants the seeds of success for the following week's group, as well as for the child in the intervening week. It is highly structured, much more so than the separate children's and parents' groups. There are four stylized, ritualistic sections, not all of equal importance or length: (1) children's group debriefing (five minutes); (2) parents' group debriefing with children's discussion (ten to twenty minutes); (3) feedback (five minutes); and (4) the selection of projects for the coming week (five to fifteen minutes).

Children's Group Debriefing

First comes a short debriefing of the children's activities. This has several purposes, some rather mundane: to give the children a chance to ventilate their enthusiasm about what they had done so they are not inclined to feel impatient and frustrated during the rest of the session; to satisfy the parents' curiosity about what the children had been doing in a way that might prevent intrusiveness and interrogation later; to let the parents know the serious intent and purpose of what the children do in their activities; to help the children realize that they have been doing something worthwhile even though they have been having fun (in other words, fun things can be useful and constructive, or conversely, useful, good things can be fun); and to give the children some further practice in reciting in a group. The debriefing in the following transcript is longer than usual because of some interesting variations that cropped up:

Dr. M.: Now what do we do? [Hands up; Mike's first.] Mike?

Mike: We tell what we did in the gym.

Dr. M.: OK, who wants to report? We have three hands up. Deanna, you were first.

Deanna: We rolled on a mat—turned somersaults—then crawled through two inner tubes, crawled across a rug, jumped rope, and then hopped around orange cones and back, and then went on scooter boards to the wall and back to the inner tubes.

Dr. M.: Very good. And what is that called?

Deanna: Obstacle course.

Dr. M.: (*to other children*) Did she miss anything? [Children shake heads.] Was it in the right order? Did she tell it in the right order? [Several children nod or say "yes."]

Dr. M.: Why was that important? Can any of the kids tell me the purpose of the activity?

George: We worked together in some way.

Dr. M.: Good.

George: We didn't race each other. [Dr. M. looks puzzled.]

Dr. A.: (*to Dr. M.*) I think George is pointing out that instead of competing, they improved their own performance. We adults who were there watching could see the improvement in each kid each time they went through the obstacle course. Like some of the kids were having trouble jumping rope at first; they got better as they went. They were able to slither through the inner tubes easier, and they got more adept at the scooter board or hopping around the red cones. Each kid was able to improve on his or her own previous performance. I think some of the kids noticed, too; they noticed it themselves.

Dr. M.: (*to Vince*) You had your hand up for something.

Vince: [Repeats sequence of activities reported by Deanna.]

Dr. M.: Very good. You also got them in the right order.

Dr. A.: I was wondering if the kids can tell the purpose of the gym activities. [Several hands up.]

Dr. M.:   (*to Mike*) Go ahead.

Mike: The purpose of it is to cooperate on something.

Dr. A.:   Cooperation, working together as a team. That's good. Anything else?

Jim: Not booing.

Dr. A.:   Not booing? You mean like if somebody kind of goofs up on it, you wouldn't make fun; is that it? [Jim nods.] Good. That's part of team work, part of working together. I actually saw some kids helping other kids, showing them how to do things. Doug showed Dave [three years old] some things. Vince showed somebody some things; a lot of kids were helping others, showing others how to do things. Another thing besides getting people to work together better is that you got parts of your own body working together, didn't you? Can you think of some of the parts of your own body working together? [Doug's hand up.] Doug?

Doug: Your heart.

Dr. A.:   Your heart? I hadn't thought about that one, but I guess it's true. OK, what else?

Doug: Your brain.

Dr. A.:   You get your brain working together with what else?

Deanna: Parts of your body like the muscles.

Dr. A.:   (*nodding*) You got your brain and your muscles working together. How did your brain know what to tell your muscles to do?

Deanna: It was thinking.

Dr. A.:   And how did it know what to think? [Vince's hand goes up.] OK, Vince?

Vince: From your eyes.

Dr. A.:   Right. You could see what you're supposed to do. And what else?

Vince: From your reflexes.

Dr. A.:   From your reflexes, good. Is there anyway else you knew what you were supposed to do with that obstacle course? If you just came down and looked at that obstacle course, would you know?

George: By hearing!

Dr. A.:   Right. You had to listen to the directions. You got your ears and your eyes and your brain and your muscles, all those things, working together. And we could see that they were working together better by the end of the time because everybody was doing a better job.

Sharing the Secret Socratically

The second segment is ostensibly sharing with the children what happened in the parents' group. This is partly to preserve a semblance of fairness after the children have reported what they did in their group (even more of what they did in their group will be made known to their parents in the feedback segment) and partly to entice the children's interest since they are often curious about what their parents talk about separately. They often rightly suspect that their parents have been talking about them. Some of the things the parents say are not suitable to share with the children, but others are relevant as topics for Socratic discussion.

By Socratic discussion we mean interacting with the children through questions in such a way that they are led into giving useful answers and are reinforced for them. This not only provides more experience in successful reciting but also demonstrates to the children and their parents how sensible they can be. Further, it provides opportunity for peer persuasion and support among the children and for appropriate consultation with parents. It demonstrates for parents how sensible the children can be when appropriately supported with respect for their opinions.

This segment is perhaps the most taxing ten or twenty minutes of the entire group and calls on all of the mental health skills of the group leader. It has to thread a line between preaching and permissiveness, between ignoring parents and kowtowing to them, between excessive seriousness and mockery, between unclarity of identification model and metamessage on the one hand and failure to respect deviant opinion and values on the other.

The following topics repeatedly occurring in the parents' group are appropriate for taking up with the children: responsibility, authority, expectation, love and liking, anger and handling of it, excuses, punishment, motivation, self-esteem, compliments and criticism, cooperation, lying, stealing, competitiveness, aggression, name calling, and apologies.

The basic format for introduction is something like this: "Well, you kids have been telling your parents about what you did in your group. Now I guess it's time to tell you about something that happened in the parents' group. One of the things that they were talking about that I think would be important to you kids is love. Who can tell me what love is?" It is important to introduce the topic and questions about it in an impersonal or abstract way to prevent defensiveness by the children, who may expect to be blamed. If the children perceive the group leader as an inquisitor for the parents, the discussion will abort. Definition questions seem the safest and most productive initial approach.

Each child is given a chance to express an opinion on each question about the topic. Sometimes this goes in order around the room, but ordinarily several hands shoot up, and it is usually advisable to take first the ones who volunteer and then fill in with direct questions to the less eager members. Eventually those who were at first less eager become more enthusiastic as they see the volunteers being reinforced for their opinions with attention and occasional words of praise.

There is vicarious reinforcement of appropriate assertiveness, thinking, articulating, and hand raising (rather than calling out) when one wishes to speak. Interruptions of the speaker are not tolerated and rarely occur as long as the group leader is sharp in noticing each child's hand and giving a chance to speak within a reasonable time.

Much of the style of this discussion is similar to William Glasser's "class meetings," including attention to having everyone visible within the circle.[1] It differs from his model in dealing with very relevant immediate concerns that the leader has gleaned from the parents and in the utilization of peer pressure to change a deviant child's opinion in a nonthreatening way. The latter is usually accomplished by asking the opinions of every child in the room, which usually results in the majority's taking a reasonable stand, and then quoting the "vote": "Let's see now, that makes five kids who think that parents should decide the time you come in at night and one kid who thinks that the kids should decide it." At this point, children with a deviant opinion usually will change to conform to the majority. If they do not, a gentle hint can be dropped: "Tom, I guess you're the only one who thinks that kids should be the ones to decide." If this does not elicit a retraction, they can be respectfully asked to give reasons for their opinion, other children can be invited to query them about it, or a direct invitation can be made to the youngsters to discuss it with each other and arrive at a unanimous agreement. Most of the children, with the example having been set by the leader, are gently supportive in their attempts to win over the deviant child and generally successful.

Rarely do children hold out in a deviant opinion, especially when they see that the group leader is willing to allow them to hold out. On several occasions, as we have acknowledged the intractability of a child's position and begun to move on to other matters, the deviant youngster hurries to conform.

Another important feature of this discussion is the recruitment of another child's parents to support a given child, as well as the recruitment of the child's own parent as a consultant, who is demonstrated thereby to the child to be an important resource person.

Examples of this Socratic discussion are found throughout part II.

Formal Feedback

Feedback is provided throughout the group to both parents and children in the form of reinforcements of constructive action and words and in the form of reflection of ideas that they bring up. The idea of feedback is so important that it is enshrined in a special section of the last parent-child segment. Star charts are used to provide the children feedback on their performance during the separate children's group and on a few items from other parts of the group. It is usually introduced by eliciting an explanation from the children of what feedback is. This may be couched in terms of the veterans explaining to the new kids or may be merely a direct question memory test.

Dr. A.: OK, what comes next?

Tom: We pick projects for next week.

Dr. A.: Before that.

Dick: We have feedback.

Dr. A.: Can you explain for the new kids what feedback is?

Dick: You get stars for the things you did right.

Dr. A.: That's right, that's positive feedback, good feedback: when you're told what things you did right. Is there another kind of feedback?

Harry: The things you did wrong or didn't do.

Dr. A.: That's right, there are two kinds of feedback: the things you did right and the things you did wrong or didn't do that you should have. We call that positive feedback and negative feedback. Why is it important to have both kinds?

Harry: So that you'll know what you did right and you can keep doing it.

Dr. A.:   That's right. But what about the negative feedback, the things you did not do or did wrong? Maybe Harriet can guess at that.

Harriet: So you won't do them anymore?

Dr. A.:   That's right. If you don't know what things you did wrong, you won't know that you should stop doing them, so you need negative feedback to know what you should stop doing. OK, so we need both positive and negative feedback, and Mrs. S. gives you both kinds. So she'll start telling you now. Go ahead, Mrs. S.

As each child's name is called, his or her chart is held up and the child is told item by item how she or he did. The children get stars for the items that they did well and check marks for those that they did partially. For the things that they failed on, there is no mark made on the chart, but a comment is made in a matter-of-fact way that they did not do it. The items listed on the star chart are: (1) walks with group (stays with group to and from gym); (2) sits quietly during directions; (3) follows directions; (4) calms self; (5) special project (for example, saying something nice to peer during children's group); (6) cooperates; (7) remembers activity or purpose of activity and shares it; (8) is helpful; (9) keeps hands and legs to self; (10) asks permission; (11) participates in group discussion; (12) reports project; (13) picks project. For partial performance such as walks with group to gym but not back, a check mark is given. This number of items ensures that every child experiences success on at least one item and no children find a clean sweep so easy that they lose interest. For a clean sweep, applause is given. For reasonable performance short of a clean sweep, verbal congratulations are given.

If time permits, the children are asked to guess how they did on each of the items before seeing the chart. They are reinforced for accurate assessment of their own performance even if the performance itself was poor. The value of being able to see oneself the way others see you is stressed.

Project Picking

This last part of the group is one of the most important because it sends the children off with a positive attitude and a specific plan for improving their behavior in the coming week. As with each other section of the group, the ritualized beginning is to ask, "What comes next?" Almost always at least one child volunteers, using one of the three words *assignment, project,* or *homework.* The children often use the word *homework,* but the group leader should not initiate the word because for some children it may carry negative connotations.

The next question is, "Who wants to go first?" Usually two or three hands shoot up, and it is important for the group leader to be watching closely enough to detect the one that is a split second sooner than the others and then to take the others in the order that they went up. Sometimes the leader has to act like an umpire who calls the close ones with the authority of absolute power. If there is enough time in a slowly paced group (usually when there are only a small number of children), it might be desirable to take the occasion to teach the children some ways of deciding on turns, such as by flipping a coin, going "eeny meeny miny moe," or "one potato, two potato, three potato." Many disordered children have not learned or have not accepted such ritualistic ways of resolving differences but often will adopt them after experiencing them in this environment. If someone has been promised a first turn because of being a loser in a tie at the reporting at the beginning of the group, this promise would preempt the other ways of deciding who gets the first turn this time.

Time is taken with each child to formulate a goal and then a plan. It is emphasized repeatedly that no matter how good a goal is, it is not likely to be attained unless the child figures out how to do it or at least how to remember it. Devising a clever plan can become a group project, with suggestions and assistance from other children as well as the child's own parent and sometimes other parents. Each child is reinforced for any efforts to be helpful to the child who is planning a project at that moment. This is done verbally not only by the group leader but also by the star chart keeper in a silent but obvious way with nonverbal display to the child.

The following is a transcript of a fairly smooth project-picking section from one group. More grueling or unusual examples can be found in the following chapter.

Dr. A.:   OK. I think Ned had his hand up first, then Ted, Korry, Eugene, and Theresa.

Ned: I'm going to work on my mathematics, learn my tables.

Dr. A.:   That's pretty tough, learning the times tables. The nice thing about it is once you learn them, you always use them. What's your plan for learning them?

Ned: Every night I'm gonna practice them so I don't flunk out of school.

Dr. A.:   OK, your goal is to learn your times tables, and your plan is to practice every night for how long? Ten minutes a night? Or could we set a mastery standard, so that every night you learn two multiplications that you didn't know before? [Ned nods.] I mean both forward and backward. Here's a tip: the big mistake is that people only learn them forward. You need to learn them backward, too. [Ned nods.] OK, Ted, you're next.

Ted: My goal is not to stutter. [He actually mumbles but calls it stuttering.]

Dr. A.:   Your goal is to keep from stuttering. What is your plan?

Ted: I'm going to clear my throat before I talk.

Dr. A.:   That's a good plan. Your goal is to keep from stuttering, and your plan is to clear your throat before you talk. OK, Korry, you're next.

Korry: My goal is to wash my hands before I eat.

Dr. A.:   OK, what's your plan for doing that? [Korry looks puzzled.] How about when you see the clean plate, you'll remember to have clean hands?

Korry: Well, how about if I see a clean table?

Dr. A.:   OK, so your goal is to wash your hands before you eat, and your plan is that when you see a clean table, you'll remember to get clean hands. OK, Eugene, are you next?

Eugene: My goal is to do my chores, and my plan is to make a list of them.

Dr. A.:   OK, your goal is to do your chores, and your plan is to make a list of them. Are you going to make the list yourself?

Eugene: Yes.

Dr. A.:   How are you going to know if you have everything on the list?

Eugene: (*grinning*) I'll get my brother to do it.

Dr. A.:   How are you going to get him to do it?

Eugene: I don't know.

Dr. A.: Will he do it if you tell him? [Eugene shrugs.] I don't think it's a good idea to pick a project where you have to make somebody else do something. It's a good idea to pick something you can do yourself. So can you agree on a list with your mother and father? Maybe you can write them down and check with your mother or father and maybe (*looking at parents*) you can agree with your mother and father that once you do everything on the list, they don't give you something else to do, right? [Eugene's mother and father nod.] Theresa, you're next.

Theresa: My goal is to stop fighting with my brother and sister, and my plan is to stop screaming.

Dr. A.: Can you hear yourself screaming? [Theresa nods.] That's good because many people can't hear themselves screaming. Maybe your mother can help you by telling you that you're screaming. Will you stop if she tells you? [Theresa nods.] Maybe it would be good if your mother had a secret signal to let you know you're screaming, like putting her hand over her mouth. Ned, did you have an idea?

Ned: Yeah, maybe her mother can give her a funny look.

Dr. A.: That's a good idea. The main thing is for mom and Theresa to agree on a signal [which they quickly do].

At the end of the project picking, an explicit statement is made that the group has ended. The new family is asked to have a seat in the waiting room so that they can be seen individually after the staff debriefing. The other families are asked if they need to be seen for anything individually such as to have a prescription rewritten and, if so, are asked to have a seat in the waiting room. (Ordinarily no one except the new family needs to be seen individually.)

Note

1. William Glasser, *Schools Without Failure* (New York: Harper and Row, 1969).

6
Project Choosing

Each child seasons the group experience to his or her own taste by choosing a project (goal and plan) to work on during the intervening week. Although technically part of the final parent-child segment, project picking is so important that we are devoting a separate chapter to it.

Basic Guidelines

As much as possible, the project should come spontaneously from the child, and it usually does. A child who has difficulty thinking of a goal is encouraged to use the parent as a consultant. When a parent wants to dictate the project with no input from the child, the group leader must firmly limit this, pointing out that it is the child's project. If the parent also wishes to take a project, that is acceptable. Sometimes there have been good results when the parents pick a simultaneous project focused on a problem that the parent has defined but that the child does not wish to consider.

In the rare instances where the child cannot or will not choose a project even with suggestions from the parent or other group members, as may happen with an oppositional five-year-old, the parent can choose the project for the child; the child can be informed gently but firmly that he or she will have an opportunity the next time to pick it. A more usual compromise is for the parent to suggest two or three things and let the child choose among them. Almost never does the group leader have to suggest a project, but this would be preferable to letting the child leave without a project.

The project needs to be something attainable. Some children their first time or two enthusiastically decide that they will pick something like, "To do everything Mommy and Daddy tell me to do." This kind of goal should be whittled down to something possible like, "To do everything Mommy and Daddy tell me between the time I get up and the time I leave for school," or "To do one thing each day that Mommy and Daddy tell me."

The goal needs to be something that the child is not already doing satisfactorily. This is one of the few reasons for a parent to veto a project. Some children, eager to have a good report, will choose something they are already doing, and it is acceptable for parents to point this out. In this case, the leader should require the child to pick a project that will involve doing something different.

The project needs to be something worthwhile in terms of self-improvement. This need not be something onerous. An acceptable project might be to make a new friend. Even the boy who decides that he will organize his baseball cards that week may be taking the first step toward organizing his life in general. If he repeatedly wants to organize his baseball cards or one week wants to organize his baseball cards, the next week organize his super hero cards, and the third week organize his rock collection, he should be nudged into something more challenging, perhaps organizing his homework or chores.

Plans assuming parental support need to be cleared with parents. Especially if the plan involves getting a reward, the parents need to be willing to supply the reward. They usually are willing but must be asked.

Repeat each child's goal and plan so that the whole group can witness the child's agreement and commitment to it and so the children can hear that you respect what they say enough to repeat it, as if it's a pearl of genius.

Transcript Examples

The best way to understand this part of the group is to sit in on several sessions. The next best is to review some transcripts of actual project picking. The transcript at the end of chapter 5 was selected for its succinctness and smooth flow. Even though it may appear contrived, it is an actual transcript and not unusual once the first few group members have been trained to set an example for new patients as they enter. Nevertheless, other aspects of project choosing need to be demonstrated. The following four transcripts illustrate various techniques, problems, and deviations in process or group development. While reviewing them, note how flexible the basic structure can be when uprising problems or therapeutic opportunities require it.

Multiple Goals and Group Planning

In this first example, four of the children had worked up to the point of being allowed several simultaneous goals, even though the usual policy emphasized one goal at a time. Note how Carl, not yet ready for multiple goals, is firmly prevented from being pressured by peer example and maternal suggestion into biting off too much. This transcript also illustrates how the group can help each child formulate a plan.

Jamie: I'm going to flush the commode each time and not touch the stereo.

Dr. A.: Your first goal is to flush the commode each time; your second goal is to leave the stereo alone. You need a plan for each one of those. [Jamie looks puzzled.] Maybe someone can help you with some ideas, and then you can pick the plan you like. The plan is how you're going to remember it.

Jeff: Maybe his mother can tell him to flush the toilet.

Dr. A.: Your idea is to have somebody remind him. Usually it's better for a kid to figure out a way to remember himself, for two reasons. First, there might not be somebody there to remind you, and the other thing is, some kids don't like it when somebody tells them to do something. They think they're being nagged.

Chuck's mother: Maybe he can write himself a note and leave it where he can see it.

Dr. A.: You're suggesting a sign? OK. So you put a sign on the inside of the bathroom door to flush the commode before leaving.

Jamie: And a sign on my door about the stereo.

Dr. A.: You put a sign on your own room door to leave the stereo alone?

Jamie: I'm going to keep a checklist to keep track.

Dr. A.: Good. Keep track. That's good. [Jeff's hand goes up.] Jeff?

Jeff: He should put a sign over the stereo instead of putting it in his room.

Dr. A.: (*turning to Jamie*) What do you think about that? Is that better?

Jamie's mother: The door is right, because the first thing he does when he gets up is go out to the stereo.

Dr. A.:	So he had the right idea putting it on the door? He knows himself! OK. That's very good, Jamie; you had yourself figured out. [Kim's hand goes up.] Kim.
Kim:	I'm going to continue with what I did last time, working on the six chores and using the list to keep track.
Dr. A.:	I was really worried about that. You did very well with them, but I wouldn't have guessed that anybody would have been able to do all that: six different things at once. So you're all set. Who's next? Was it Karen [Kim's sister] that was next?
Karen:	I'm going to do my six chores again, too.
Dr. A.:	This time you got a little over half. Are you going to set some mark? Are you going to try doing like 60 percent of them?
Karen:	And something else.
Dr. A.:	You want to do something besides the six things that mom tells you to do? What is it?
Karen:	I want to work on cleaning up my room and keeping it neat by putting stuff back when I'm done with it.
Dr. A.:	So your goal is to keep your room cleaned up, and your plan is that whenever you take something out, you put it back away when you're through with it. That sounds very good. All right. I guess Dan is next.
Dan:	She can try to cut her misses down to 25 percent.
Dr. A.:	Can we put that the other way? That she brings the good days to 75 percent? We'll try to concentrate on the good part. [Carl's hand goes up.] Carl?
Carl:	I'll brush my teeth.
Dr. A.:	Is that what you want to take for your project? [Carl nods.] Dan was ahead of you.

Dan:	I want to do my chore list again.
Dr. A.:	You're going to keep the same goal. Are you going to have a different plan or the same one?
Dan:	Same plan.
Dr. A.:	OK. Are you going to set a different—like you got half this time—are you going to try for 60 percent or something like that?
Dan:	Yes, and Mom said she'd give me ice cream if I do it 75 percent of the time.
Dr. A.:	So that's your incentive, then. You have kind of a new plan: you're going to think about the ice cream you're going to get if you can improve your performance. Good. Now, Carl, we're ready for you.
Carl:	I'm going to brush my teeth. [Carl's mother shakes her head no and interrupts, indicating he does it already.]
Dr. A.:	Oh. You're already brushing your teeth. That's great; you're already doing that. Now can you pick something that you're not already doing. What is it? [Carl stares blankly.]
Dr. A.:	You can get some help from your mother. It's all right to talk with her and get some help on it. (*turning to his mother*) Maybe you could give him a couple of choices, and maybe he can pick one of them.
Carl's mother:	Maybe he can clear the table where he sits or feed the dog.
Carl:	I'll clear my spot.
Dr. A.:	So your goal is to clean your spot off the table after you are finished eating supper?
Carl:	And feed the dog.
Dr. A.:	You only have to pick one thing. What's your plan for remembering? How will you remember to clean your spot off?

Carl:	My mother will tell me.
Dr. A.:	Your mother would remind you?
Carl:	Yeah.
Dr. A.:	Maybe the other kids have some ideas how you can remember yourself. It's a lot more fun if you remember yourself, instead of having your mother tell you. Most kids don't like to have their mothers telling them things all the time. [Dan's hand goes up.] Dan has an idea.
Dan:	He can put a note to remind himself.
Dr. A.:	So you could put a note next to where he sits at the table. Do you know how to read, Carl? Maybe just seeing the piece of paper would remind you.
Jeff:	He could make a picture.
Dr. A.:	That's right. Good. You can read a picture, can't you? That's good thinking, Jeff. Kim has an idea, too. What is it?
Kim:	He could put a note under his plate.
Dr. A.:	So it could be like a place mat. He could put a piece of paper under his plate and it would help to catch anything that would fall off, and also seeing it there would remind him to clean it up. You could use newspaper for the place mat, and then you could throw it away each time.
Carl:	My mother could check it each time.
Dr. A.:	OK. You can call your mother over to check it to see what a good job you did each time. That would help, wouldn't it? [Carl is obviously so dependent that he must include his mother somehow, so Dr. A. frames a compromise in which Carl can feel some maternal presence but still operate on his own initiative.] OK, Jeff, you need to take a project.
Jeff:	I am going to stay at the table during dinner.

Dr. A.:	OK, your goal is staying at the table during the meal, and your plan for remembering it is what? [Jeff looks puzzled. Carl's hand goes up.] OK, Carl, do you have an idea?
Carl:	He could stay at the table and don't talk with his mouth full.
Dr. A.:	OK. He would think about getting his mouth empty before he leaves. He would have to swallow everything first. [Jeff nods assent.] Who's next? Peter?
Peter:	I'm going to help clear the table every night and do it before Dad tells me to.
Dr. A.:	OK. Your goal is to keep your dad from having to tell you to clean the table off, and your plan is to hurry up and do it before he can tell you. That sounds good. Ed, did you pick yours yet? I don't believe you did.
Ed:	Go to bed on time and watch TV before 9 o'clock.
Dr. A.:	So your goal is to go to bed on time; your plan is that you get ready for bed and watch a TV program that goes off at 9. [Ed nods.] That sounds very good.

Most of the kids were able to say their goal and plan very quickly, and they got stars for that. I'm really impressed with how well you kids did today. Seems like people are really trying to help each other, and that's nice to see. Congratulations to all of you.

Oppositional and Passive Project Picking

Ordinarily most of the children are enthusiastic about picking their projects, and practically all are cooperative. Occasionally a child may be reticent or even oppositional. Most such incidents involve preschoolers and may become a concern to other children. In such cases, it may be useful to ascribe the behavior to immaturity, which reassures all the children that the behavior will improve and provides a face-saving rationale for the aberrant child to begin conforming. We usually leave a child suspected to be oppositional until toward the end to ensure that the others get their fair share of time and attention and let them set a good example, which is often followed. The following transcript cuts into the middle of a project shoosing session. Four-year-old Frank has been oppositional in a previous session.

Donna: I'm gonna do my chores without whining or crying.

Dr. A.: You put a nice condition on there: that you are going to do them without whining or crying. That's good.

Donna: Yeah, and I'm gonna check them off when I do them.

Dr. A.: OK, and when you feel like whining or crying, you'll think about how nice it'll be to check that thing off on the list. Right? Good. OK, we have Frank, Greg, and Ed. [Greg's hand goes up.] OK, we're ready for you, Greg.

Greg: Keep my room clean.

Dr. A.: You're going to keep your room clean. OK, what's your plan for remembering that?

Greg: I don't know.

Dr. A.: OK, maybe some people here can help you. Who can help Greg? His goal is to keep his room clean, and he needs a plan for remembering to do that. Who can help him to do that?

Konrad: Pick up the things you see in your room.

Dr. A.: What do you think about that, Konrad's idea? That every time you see something on the floor, you pick it up. [Greg nods.] You like that idea? Oh, Doug has an idea too.

Doug: Like when you are in your room, you can just pick out one thing at a time.

Dr. A.: OK, if you would just take one thing out at a time, then it is not too hard to put away. [Greg nods enthusiastically.] You like that idea. OK, so you have two plans. Your goal is to keep your room clean, your plan is to put things away whenever you see anything on the floor, and also to just take one toy at a time out to play with. OK, let's see. [Ed's hand goes up.] Ok, Ed. What's your goal?

Ed:	My goal is to come in at 8:00.
Dr. A.:	To come in at 8:00. OK, and your plan?
Ed's mother:	That's not a problem.
Dr. A.:	Oh, it's not? OK, you should pick something that is going to be different from what you have been doing—like if you've been forgetting to brush your teeth, and you start brushing your teeth.
Ed:	Keep my room clean.
Dr. A.:	OK, you're going to keep your room clean. And what's your plan? How will you remember to keep it clean?
Ed:	I'm gonna put my things away where they belong.
Dr. A.:	OK, how are you going to remember to do that? [Ed looks puzzled.] Doug has an idea to help.
Doug:	Like when you take something out, you put it right back where it belongs, unless you're wearing it. [Ed nods.]
Dr. A.:	All right, so your goal is to keep your room clean, and your plan is whenever you take anything out, put it right back again if you're not going to be wearing it. OK, let's see. We have Frank yet. [Four-year-old Frank and eight-year-old Terry have been playing on the floor, quietly at first. At this point Frank becomes belligerent and punches at Terry, who seems surprised and disappointed.] Frank, can you get away from Terry long enough to pick your project?
Frank:	(*belligerently*) No!
Dr. A.:	First you need a goal.
Frank's mother:	What are you going to do? You told me.
Frank:	I don't know.
Dr. A.:	You want your mother to tell it?
Frank:	No.

Dr. A.:	Now, you remember how this works: either you tell it, or your mother tells it.
Frank:	No!
Dr. A.:	Well, it doesn't work that way. So we're going to have your mother go ahead and tell it.
Frank:	No!
Frank's mother:	He's going to pick up his toys and . . .
Frank:	No! [Frank starts screaming and pouting.]
Konrad:	(*hand up*) I know.
Dr. A.:	Oh, Konrad heard it. OK, you want to tell it, Konrad? [Terry is trying to console and soothe Frank, who requites with slapping and kicking.] Terry, just leave him alone. When a kid is screaming or pouting, you just leave him alone. All right, Konrad.
Konrad:	He said that he was going to put all of his toys away.
Dr. A.:	He was going to put all of his toys away.
Frank:	(*screaming*) No!
Dr. A.:	(*ignores*) OK, and what was his plan for remembering that?
Konrad:	I didn't hear a plan.
Dr. A.:	Oh, you didn't hear the plan. (*turning to mother*) Do you know the plan?
Frank's mother:	To remind him when he is finished playing to put them away.
Dr. A.:	OK, you're to remind him about it. You'll help him with his plan? [Mother nods.] OK, that's all right. (*to Frank*) It's OK to ask your mother or father to help you with a plan like that, but the idea is usually you remember some-

thing yourself. [Frank has become nastier with Terry, who is looking disappointed that he cannot soothe Frank.] OK, Terry, I think you better get away from him, or first thing you know he might hurt you, and then you would get mad. It's better to just get away from him. When somebody plays nasty, just leave them alone. There's no point in trying to play with someone who is going to try to hurt you. [Terry pulls back five feet, and Dr. A. continues.] Have you ever seen anyone act like that before? Who has seen anyone pout before? [Several hands up.] Who has ever acted that way yourself when you were younger? [All staff hands up; most parents' and children's hands up.] Frank is only four years old and still needs to learn some things about behaving. Maybe he can learn from you older kids. [Frank settles down during this discussion.]

The following week, Frank was able to report with pride that he had put his toys away six days out of seven. The next transcript shows Frank's project picking behavior at the end of that group.

Marathon Mentor

Most project picking sessions flow well enough to be concluded within ten or fifteen minutes. An occasional one, though, taxes the leader's stamina. The following transcript illustrates one of the more difficult marathons. One of the factors prolonging it was the attendance of eight families, which stretches the upper limits of the group's elastic structure. On high attendance days, extra time should be reserved for project picking. Even so, it is sometimes necessary to extend the group to give everyone an adequate opportunity. This transcript, taken a week after the preceding transcript, also provides follow-up on Frank.

Dr. A.:	Who wants to go first? [Four hands go up.] Nora, Konrad, Doug, and Greg, and then others. Nora, you're first. Go ahead.
Nora:	My plan is to come in and go to bed on time.
Dr. A.:	OK, you're going to come in and go to bed on time. That's your goal. How are you going to remember to do that?
Nora:	Look at the clock.

Dr. A.:   Do you have a clock with you all the time wherever you are?

Nora: No.

Dr. A.:   Well, how are you going to do that, then? Maybe somebody else has an idea. How could she remember to come in on time? [No response; turning back to Nora] What time are you supposed to come in?

Nora: Dark.

Dr. A.:   When you see it's starting to get dark. [Doug's hand goes up.] Doug has an idea.

Doug: When the shadows get real long, she can come in.

Konrad: She can look at the clock, or if she's at a friend's, ask the friend to check.

Dr. A.:   Dave has an idea, too. What is it Dave?

Dave: When she sees a little bit of darkness in the sky.

Dr. A.:   OK, when you see a little bit of darkness in the sky. So three different people had ideas. Which one of those do you like?

Nora: Dave's.

Dr. A.:   And what one was that? [Nora mumbles.] Can you say it again? [Dave repeats it.] Can you say it now yourself? I think you should pick one you can say yourself. If you can't say it yourself, you probably won't remember it.

Nora: I'll ask my friend to look at her clock.

Dr. A.:   So your goal is to come in when it starts getting dark and go to bed, and your plan is to ask a friend to check the time if you're at their house or if you're at your own house to come in and look at the clock yourself.

Joe: What if she's not at anybody's house?

Dr. A.:	Well, how could she tell what time it's getting to be on the street?
Joe:	Street lights.
Dr. A.:	OK, that was a good idea: remember when the street lights come on. Can you use that if you're out on the street? [Nora nods.] So your plan is if you're out at a friends house or your own house, you look at the clock; if you're out on the street, you come in when the street lights come on. I think Konrad was next.
Konrad:	My goal is to come in when the street lights come on.
Dr. A.:	Your goal is to come in when you should come in. When the street lights come on; that's your plan, too, isn't it? To come in when the street lights come on. So your goal is to come in on time, and your plan is to notice when the street lights come on. That's your signal to get in the house. All right, Doug.
Doug:	My goal is to get up when I'm called.
Dr. A.:	Your goal is to get up when you're called, and your plan is what? Anybody want to help him with the plan? Doug needs a plan to remember to get up in the morning as soon as he is called.
Greg:	Think about the things you have to do.
Doug:	I know! I can count to ten.
Dr. A.:	Kind of have a countdown, like a rocket blasting off. Maybe you should count backwards: 10, 9, 8, 7 . . . and you jump out of bed and it's a blast-off. That sounds good. So you have your goal and plan. Greg is next.
Greg:	(*mumbles*)
Dr. A.:	Your goal is to do what?
Greg:	Clean the kitchen.

Dr. A.:	And how are you going to remember? Do you want some help from the other kids? [Greg nods.] OK, who can help Greg remember? His goal is to clean the kitchen. He needs a plan for remembering. Nora.
Nora:	Clean the living room.
Dr. A.:	What? His goal is to clean the kitchen. [Doug's hand goes up.] Doug, you have an idea?
Doug:	First he can clear the dishes off the table, then wipe the table.
Dr. A.:	That's kind of organizing the work—how he's going to clean the kitchen. OK. But how is he going to remember to get started on that? Here's a suggestion: when the meal is over. That would remind you to clean the kitchen. Would that work? [Greg nods.] One thing I'm going to ask you. Is it something you're not doing already? [Greg mumbles.] Pardon?
Greg:	Yesterday.
Dr. A.:	Well, this should be something you're not already doing. Are you already doing it every day? Are you or not?
Greg:	I did yesterday.
Dr. A.:	But are you already cleaning the kitchen? Yesterday you did once, but how about most of the time?
Greg:	No.
Dr. A.:	You don't do it most of the time? [Greg shakes head.] You're not already doing it most of the time. So your goal is to do it now. Your plan is after each meal you think about cleaning it up.
Greg:	I'll make a chart.
Dr. A.:	You can check it off each time you do it, can't you? Keep a record and report back. Now who was next? I think that was all the hands. Dave?

Dave:	I'll stay at the table the whole meal.
Dr. A.:	Your goal is to stay at the table for the whole meal. OK, and what is your plan?
Dave:	Remember that I'm there to eat and not to play.
Dr. A.:	Your plan is to remember that the purpose of sitting at the table is to eat. OK, so your goal is to stay at the table for the whole meal, and your plan is to remember the purpose of sitting there and maybe think about dessert. OK, who's next? Donna, are you ready?
Donna:	I'm going to stop goofing off.
Dr. A.:	Your goal is to stop goofing off. What do you mean by goofing off? [Donna's mother starts to answer.] Why don't we see if Donna can explain it, and if you want to add something afterward . . .
Donna:	Once I went off and watched a movie on TV when I should have cleaned my room.
Dr. A.:	Oh, you went off and watched a movie instead of doing your job. So your goal really is to do the thing you're told rather than watching a movie or something else. Now, how many things a day are you going to do right away without goofing off? This could turn out to be a never-ending job. You could be doing this all day, and you could give up on it. I want you to pick out how many things a day you're going to do that way.
Donna:	Five.
Dr. A.:	You think it should be five times. [Konrad raises his hand.] You had an idea, Konrad?
Konrad:	She could try and see how quickly she can do it and time herself.
Dr. A.:	That sounds like a good idea.
Greg's mother:	Two or three things a day should be plenty.

Dr. A.: The suggestion from Greg's mother was two or three a day. (*to Donna*) And I think you have kind of agreed with that. Is that enough to suit you, Donna? And your mother makes the list of things? So your goal is to do two or three things a day that your mother tells you without goofing off, and your plan is your mother will make the list, and you will check the list to see what you're supposed to do. OK. Now let's see . . . we still have Frank and Mort. Just two left. Frank, are you ready? [Four-year-old Frank had been oppositional in the past.] There are two ways to do it. You can pick the project yourself, or your mother can pick one for you. [Frank begins a tantrum, and his mother restrains him as she had been shown in previous groups.] I guess we'll go with Rick and then come back. (*to Rick, the new child*) You can pick something that you haven't been able to do very well or something you want to learn or a new habit that you want to get into. It can be some idea that you get from your mother, but you can use your own idea. You need to have a goal and then a plan as to how you are going to do it. What would you like to do? what is your goal?

Rick: I don't know. (*turns to mother*)

Dr. A.: You want to get an idea from your mother? You can use her as a consultant. Why don't you get some ideas from her and pick one of them. She might be able to give you a couple of ideas, and you can pick which one you want. We'll go to Frank [who has settled down] and come back to you.

Frank: (*mumbles*)

Dr. A.: (*supportively*) I couldn't hear.

Frank's mother: Eat everything on his plate.

Dr. A.: Is that what you said? [Frank nods.] Eat everything on your plate. That sounds like a good idea. What is your plan for remembering to do that?

Frank: (*mumbling*) . . . go . . . 'n play . . .

Dr. A.: You get to go in your room and play after?

Frank:	. . . with shovel . . .
Dr. A.:	Play with the shovel! Go outside and dig in the sand? [Frank and his mother nod.] So your goal is to eat everything on your plate, and your plan is that after you eat, you get to go outside and dig in the sand with the shovel. Is that it? [Frank nods.] Frank, I want to congratulate you on how you settled down, and you're behaving well now. [Frank begins grinning.] You are starting to grow up, aren't you? You're acting more like the big boys. I'll bet your mother is proud of you now. Sometimes mothers and fathers get embarrassed about the way the kids act, but the other mothers and fathers and the other kids know that that's the way little kids do sometimes; you just have to help them control themselves until they get over it. Then they settle down. Rick, now we're ready for you.
Rick:	Brush my teeth.
Dr. A.:	You're going to brush your teeth; that's your goal.
Rick:	And brush my hair . . . and wash my face.
Dr. A.:	Oh, brush your teeth, comb your hair, and wash your face. That's really three things. Usually people pick one thing for a project. You want to try all three? [Nods.] You're going to do it all together at the same time? [Nods.] OK. How are you going to remember to do that? [Rick looks puzzled.] Let's get some ideas from the other kids.
Dave:	When he goes to the bathroom.
Dr. A.:	When you have to go to the bathroom—that would remind you? OK. That's where you wash your face, comb your hair, brush your teeth, isn't it? [Doug's hand goes up.]
Doug:	Everybody has to go to the bathroom in the morning.
Dr. A.:	How about that: you have to go to the bathroom in the morning; most people do, so that would work.
Konrad's mother:	After Konrad combs his hair and gets all ready for school, I let him go out to play with the other kids until the bus comes.

Dr. A.: How about that? Would that work?

Konrad's mother: Sometimes he goes out without combing his hair.

Dr. A.: Maybe you need to be careful with that because if you let him get away without doing it, then the incentive is lost for doing it.

Rick's mother: If he does it before going out, I won't have to call him back in.

Dr. A.: (*to Rick*) That's good. It would be easier for both you and your mother if you do it first, because then you don't have to come back in to do it.

Dave: (*inaudible*)

Dr. A.: I couldn't hear you.

Dave: Rick and his mother could both comb their hair and wash their faces at the same time.

Dr. A.: That's one thing. Mrs. G. had an idea.

Mrs. G.: He could leave a note on the table by his bed.

Dr. A.: Did you understand that, Rick? You could leave a note on the table for yourself. Or you could lay the comb and toothbrush someplace where you could see it when you walk in the bathroom. That's another thing. So you have a lot of ideas. Which one do you like best? Which one do you want to pick for remembering? You have the idea of leaving a note on the table, leaving a picture on the bathroom door, remembering that you can go outside and play as soon as you do those things.

Rick: I'll do it all.

Dr. A.: You want to use all those ideas? The other idea is for you and your mother to do it at the same time. Which one of those ideas do you like best? Can you remember the ideas? [Rick looks puzzled.] Name one of the ideas. [No response.] Do you want to pick somebody to say it over again so you can hear it?

Rick: Leave a note.

Dr. A.:   You're going to leave a note. So your goal is to wash your face, brush your teeth, and comb your hair in the morning. Your plan is to leave a note on the table the night before. So everybody has a project. [Whew!]

Punting

Sometimes all the king's horses and all the king's men can't get a project picked in the time available. In the well-known art of punting, one admits that scoring is impossible this time and attempts to establish a better field position for the next time. In the following transcript, five-year-old Larry has been left until last, after the others volunteered to choose projects.

Dr. A.:   OK, Larry, what do you want to work on this week? You can either pick something by yourself or ask your mother for some ideas.

Larry: (*mumbles*)

Dr. A.:   Larry, I couldn't hear.

Mrs. R.:   (*interrupts*) He wants me to do it.

Dr. A.:   (*to Larry*) Oh, you want your mother to pick something? [Larry nods.] OK, your mother can pick something, but then we'll check with you to see if it makes sense.

Mrs. R.:   I really think it's time for Larry to pick something that he can work on all by himself. I think he ought to start doing things that require a little more effort, like putting together a little more difficult puzzle, something that's a little more effort than, well . . .

Dr. A.:   You mean something like putting together a puzzle that takes ten minutes or so?

Mrs. R.:   Yes, like one with seventeen pieces, not five.

Dr. A.:   Do you have a size in between, like ten or twelve pieces?

Mrs. R.:   Yes, I think it would be good for him to put together something that requires seventeen.

Dr. A.:   OK, so he can put together a five-piece puzzle now?

Mrs. R.:   Of course. And I know he can do a seventeen-piece puzzle, but I think it's something that he needs to learn how to stay with by himself.

Dr. A.:   OK, how many different puzzles do you have? Do you have graduating sizes, like five pieces, seven pieces, ten pieces, or twelve pieces? [Mrs. R. nods.] How about this, then? (*to Larry*) The project on the first day would be to put together a six- or seven-piece puzzle; then tomorrow you could put together the six-piece puzzle again and then an eight-piece puzzle. The six- or seven-piece puzzle will be easier because you've done it already. Then the next day you can put together the eight-piece puzzle again and a ten-piece puzzle. Each day you move up one more and put together the one from the day before for practice. Larry, is that something you want to do? [Shakes head.] Then how do you want to do it? [No response.] Do you want your mother to give you another choice? Then you can pick between the two? [Larry nods.] (*to Mrs. R.*) OK, can you give Larry another idea?

Mrs. R.:   (*to Larry*) Maybe you can draw a nice picture and fill it all in so we can put it on the wall.

Dr. A.:   Oh, you can draw something or trace over it. You can either draw a whole picture so you can put it on the wall, or you can put together a harder puzzle. Which one do you want to pick?

Larry: I can't do it!

Dr. A.:   Which one can't you do?

Larry: I can't do them.

Dr. A.:   Oh. Your problem is that you think you can't do things.

Mrs. R.:   I think Larry can do things, but he needs to do things that he could find self-gratification in.

Dr. A.:   Larry, can you find one thing to work on each day that you can do yourself? [Larry looks down silently.] Maybe we need some help from the other guys. What could he do? [Fred's hand goes up.] OK, Fred?

Fred: He could go outside and do some exercises.

Larry: I can't.

Dr. A.:   (*to mother*) Do you think he could do that by himself?

Mrs. R.:   He would probably wander around. I would like it that he go all the way up to the corner and back. I've seen him do that.

Dr. A.:   OK, it sounds like Larry's problem is that he's convinced he can't do things even though other people have seen him do things. [Tim's hand goes up.] Tim, what ideas do you have about that?

Tim: He could build blocks.

Dr. A.:   OK. Have you seen him do it?

Tim: No, he wouldn't do it today.

Dr. A.:   Oh, so it kind of looks like Larry is going to pout rather than try. Fred?

Fred: Maybe he could start helping his mother do things, and then she could gradually let go. Then he could do it by himself.

Dr. A.:   That's a good idea. In fact, I think she's tried that already. That's the way any mother or father would want to do it, though. It sounds like you guys have lots of good ideas about things that Larry could do. I think the main problem is that Larry has his mind made up not to do it, and I don't know whether there's anything anybody can do to help Larry as long as he wants to pout and not try things. So you've given lots of good ideas, and I guess the rest is up to Larry, whether he is going to try something.

Have any of you guys ever done this, where you get mad and decide "I'm just not going to do anything"? Have you ever done that? [Nods from several children.] You have, Fred? [Nods.] You have, Luke? [Nods.] I guess everybody has done that some time in their life. [Fred's father raises hand.] You have too, Mr. P.?

[Laughter.] I guess I have to put my hand up too, if it comes to that. [More laughter.] I guess we'd all have to put our hand up. Part of growing up is learning that that is not much fun—refusing to do things. And I guess Larry still has to learn some of that. Time to stop for today. I'll look forward to hearing from you guys next week and how you did with your projects.

The following week Larry was cooperative enough to score on third down.

Part II
Clinical Applications
and Issues

7
A Basic Task:
Feeling Good about Yourself

Most learning- and behavior-disordered children have extremely low self-esteem and self-confidence; these self-images are partly based on reality. The children have experienced repeated failure in academic tasks, in attempts to make and keep friends, in attempts to please their parents, and in attempts to get appropriate attention. Consequently they have experienced the frustrated exasperation and even hostility of parents, teachers, and peers and have absorbed the message that they are inept schmucks. When you feel like a schmuck, you tend to act like a schmuck; it becomes a self-fulfilling prophecy.

Part of the reprogramming task is to help the children (even force them, if necessary) to stop feeling like schmucks and begin feeling competent. The competence has to be reality based, as it can be when the youngsters' other activities are programmed so that they begin experiencing success. This chapter illustrates strategies and techniques for programming the child's self-perception to match increasing competence in performance and social skills. It includes raising the parents' consciousness of the problem and modeling for them how to nurture the child's fledgling self-esteem.

Dr. A.: OK. Who wants to report on his project first? Neal, I think your hand went up just a split second before Kurt's.

Neal: I was supposed to stop yelling at my mom.

Dr. A.: OK, what was your plan? How were you going to do that?

Neal: Whenever I felt like yelling at my mom, I was gonna go to my room until I calmed myself down, and then I was gonna say how I felt to my mom instead of yelling at her.

Dr. A.: How did you do?

Neal: [Gazing sheepishly and evading eye contact, Neal muttered a few words.]

Dr. A.:   Neal, I'm not sure that anyone could hear you. Could you use your playground voice? How many times did you manage to go to your room, calm yourself down and then state how you felt so you wouldn't yell at your mom?

Neal: Not very much. [Eyes still glued to the floor.]

Stop for a minute and think how you would respond. It sounds as if the child is reporting a failure. Disordered children typically are thrown by unexpected disappointments and overwhelmed by failure. The therapist needs to model being able to take disappointments in stride, learn from mistakes, and be willing to discuss the facts of the situation without fear. This is important modeling not only for the child but for the parent. Therefore, in such a situation, it is necessary to explore courageously but gently and supportively in some such manner as the following:

Dr. A.:   You mean your plan didn't work? You still yelled at your mom? [Neal nods.] Well, what happened?

Mrs. P.: [Neal's mother, Mrs. P., had been involved in vicious cycle arguments with Neal at the time they first started the group.] Neal, now that's not the truth. Why don't you tell Dr. A. how you really did?

Neal: [No response.]

Dr. A.:   Well, maybe if Neal doesn't want to tell us, I can ask you, Mrs. P., to explain. Would it be OK with you, Neal, if your mom told us what happened?

Neal: Yes.

Mrs. P.: Neal did much better. There were times when we really could have got into it but Neal went to his room, and when he calmed down, he came out, and we had a real good discussion.

Dr. A.:   Well, that sounds like an improvement! How many times did he go to his room when he felt like yelling?

Mrs. P.: Oh, I would say just a few times.

Dr. A.:   Could you put a number on it?

Mrs. P.:   About three times.

Dr. A.:   You mean Neal improved from zero times to three times?

Mrs. P.:   Yes, that's right.

Dr. A.:   Well, I'm glad to see that the plan worked, and Neal improved. It also makes me feel good to see that you noticed Neal's improvement. But I was kind of wondering why Neal didn't say so? Did you realize, Neal, that you improved?

Note how techniques of behavior management are gradually introduced. The idea of counting, using exact numbers instead of vague generalizations, is now familiar to Mrs. P. Reinforcing Mrs. P. in front of the group will help her to become more confident in her competence as an effective mother and will help her son to see her not only in a more positive light but as someone who can learn new things as well.

Dr. A.:   OK, who's next? [Tom's hand goes up. His brother Kurt is pouting about not being first and does not bother to raise a hand. Dr. A. forgot that Kurt was to be second, with destructive consequences, as we will see.]

Tom: I was supposed to clean my room every day.

Dr. A.:   What was your plan?

Tom: I was supposed to make a chart and hang it up on my door with the days of the week on it.

Dr. A.:   OK, you were going to remind yourself to clean your room by making a chart so you could check off each day of the week. How did you do?

Kurt: Lousy! (*aggressively tattling on his brother, Tom, and still angry that he wasn't allowed to go first*) [At this point Dr. A. should have interpreted Kurt's anger but still did not remember. Instead, he merely set a limit.]

Dr. A.:   Kurt, why don't you let Tom answer for himself? Tom, how did you do?

Tom: Well, I made the chart. I got the paper from school from my teacher, and I hung it on my door.

Dr. A.: Did the chart remind you to clean your room?

Tom: (*looks spaced out*)

Kurt: Yeah, he only cleaned his room some of the time, and he filled out the chart last night. [We can see why chapter 2 cautions the group leader to remember the order of hands.]

Dr. A.: How many days did you clean your room, Tom?

Tom: Just four. [Note how Tom assumes his brother's negative attitude even though he had improved.]

Dr. A.: You cleaned your room four days out of seven! That's a great improvement from not cleaning your room at all! I bet you didn't even realize that, Tom, did you? [Tom brightens. Kurt raises his hand.] OK, Kurt, it's your turn to report. What was your assignment?

Kurt: To stop fighting with Tom.

Dr. A.: What was your plan?

Kurt: When Tom picks a fight with me, I was supposed to walk away.

Dr. A.: How did you do?

Kurt: OK, I guess.

Dr. A.: Could you be more specific? How many times?

Kurt: Well, Tom didn't pick any more fights with me. [Laughter from whole group.]

Dr. A.: None? You mean you didn't have to walk away because Tom didn't pick any fights?

Kurt: Yep.

Dr. A.: Well, maybe I better check with your mother and see if she agrees.

Mrs. F.: That's right. I don't exactly know what's come over them, but Kurt and Tom didn't get into any fights to speak of.

Dr. A.: That's really good. Maybe just by thinking about the problem behavior and figuring out a plan to change it prevents the problem for some people. Of course, it won't work that easily for everyone.

Later, at the separate parents' group:

Dr. E.: I was impressed that the children made good progress this week but some did not recognize it themselves.

Mrs. F.: It didn't seem like they did recognize. We were all more pleased, I think, than they were.

Dr. E.: I felt it was almost like pulling teeth to get them to report on how well they did.

Mrs. B.: They seem like they don't want to say good things about themselves when we're around. Maybe they would be different among themselves or if we weren't there.

Mrs. F.: Maybe they feel funny saying something good about themselves in front of the other kids, too. I think, though, with kids like ours, they are in trouble in school so much of the time that it's hard for 'em to say good things about themselves. They are not used to hearing good things said about themselves, let alone reporting it themselves.

Dr. E.: Every time one of them was asked how they did, judging by the way they appeared, I had expected them to say that they had not done so well. But it turned out that they really had done well. Perhaps in addition to what you've all said, they have a difficult time recognizing good behavior. They are not used to being successful at things a parent would normally expect of a kid. It's a new role they have to learn, to get accustomed to.

Mrs. E.: We're really proud of the way Kurt has been coming along. I think Kurt is proud of himself too. One morning this week he asked me while he was getting dressed, "Can't I ever stay home from school?" I said, "Kurt, I'll tell you that if you get all A's (which I don't think is an unreasonable goal for him), you can stay home one day and do whatever you like." I think it is possible for him now. Right now that is what he is striving for.

Later the parents and children rejoined each other:

Dr. A.: Before we talk about something very important that the parents mentioned, I would like to hear what you kids did. Neal, since this is your second time here, this would be a good chance for you to report on what the kids did. Jump in and tell your mother what you did. [Note the tactic of choosing Neal to report. Although it was a calculated risk because Neal may have refused to comment, the leader felt Neal had progressed enough in rapport and confidence to warrant the attempt to build his self-confidence in front of his peers and mother.]

Neal: We played with the parachute.

Dr. A.: Did you know how big a parachute was?

Neal: Yes.

Dr. A.: Oh, had you seen one before?

Neal: Yes, in school.

Dr. A.: What did you do with the parachute?

Neal: We played popcorn.

Dr. A.: What's that?

Neal: It's when you put two balls in it and throw it up.

Dr. A.: Oh, and make it pop! Now to make it work, could one person do that by himself?

Neal: Uh-uh.

Dr. A.: So what did you have to do to make it work?

Neal: (*counting aloud*) One, two, three, four, five . . .

Dr. A.: Right, there were five people working together. How did all five work together? You all had to do the same thing at the same time. How did you do that? [Note how the leader expands the child's thoughts.]

Neal: We counted and lifted it up.

Dr. A.:   Oh, so you got your eyes and ears working together. Before you did that, you had to listen to the directions, didn't you?

Kurt: (*indignantly*) We did that!

Dr. A.:   Then you had to remember them, and then something very important had to happen. A four-letter word—does anybody know what it is? [Laughter from some of the student doctors.] [There is no verbal response; the children sit in a trance-like mental search for the answer.] Plan! You had to plan. That's something we talk a lot about in here. You work your mind to plan something. That's what helps you do something. OK? So you had practice in planning. After you plan something, you can do it.

Before Mrs. S. gives us the feedback, I just kind of wanted to talk to you kids about something that the parents were talking about. This was something that they were wondering about. What they were wondering about was how they can get you kids to realize that you are pretty good kids, that you do good things, and even if you make a mistake, it doesn't mean that you are a bad kid. Do you guys have some ideas about this? What can be done to help you to realize that you're pretty good kids? Did you know that your parents thought you were pretty good kids?

[Note the repeated imbedding of the assumed fact, "You're pretty good kids." This hypnotic and neurolinguistic programming technique slips the desirable concept into the child's unconscious when a bald assurance would have elicited defensive disbelief.]

[The children sit in stunned attentive silence.] Don't you think that there is anything to help you realize you're good? Neal? Tom? Bob? How about you, Kurt, since you are the veteran here today, and you seem to feel good about yourself these days? What could be done to help these guys feel good about themselves?

Kurt: Drawing good.

Dr. A.:   Oh. Drawing good, but suppose they can't draw so good? What then?

Kurt: I don't know.

Dr. A.:   Well, some people are good at drawing, but others are not. Some people are good at sports; others are not. Some people are good at math; others are not. Some people are good at music; others are not. Everybody has something different that they're good at. Does that give you some ideas about how somebody can feel better about themselves?

Kurt: (*after a long pause*) They can play baseball!

Think how you would respond to this. What do you think the child meant? Did he misunderstand the question? Was he trying to obstruct? Was he a baseball lover who was getting bored with this discussion? How would you understand, interpret, and respond? A general principle in reprogramming is to interpret ambiguous statements and situations in the most favorable light, that is, the way that redounds most to the child's credit while at the same time advancing the concepts you are trying to sell.

In this case the interpretation that would seem best to accomplish that dual purpose is that the youngster was suggesting that if someone could not draw well, maybe he or she could play baseball well. Therefore, the therapist gave credit to the child for this insightful concrete example:

Dr. A.:   Right! They can find something else that they can do. Maybe it's not baseball but just something they can do pretty well. If they are having trouble at something they are not good at, they can remind themselves of something they do well, right? Are there any other ideas about what a kid can do if he feels discouraged? Maybe some of the grown-ups have some ideas.

Dr. E.:   Dr. A., maybe the kids don't have ideas about this because they don't know what they do well. Do you think that it's possible they get all confused? Maybe there are some ways they can figure that out. I wonder if the kids have trouble figuring out what they do well. Does that ever happen? Kurt? Tom? Neal? [The children look bewildered.]

Dr. A.:   Yes, that could be a problem, and maybe they are not even sure. They know that they do some things bad and some things good. Maybe they have ideas about what they do good. But maybe since they are not sure which is good and which is bad, they kind of figure everything they do is bad. Maybe they have a hard time listening when somebody tells them they do something right.

Dr. E.: Yes, that's possible. One of the things kids learn to do here is getting used to succeeding. It's sometimes even hard for some adults to get used to.

Dr. A.: How are you guys on taking compliments? If somebody says, "Hey, that's a nice job you did there, Neal; I really like that drawing" or "That was a good pitch you made" or "That was a good math paper; you got a B+ on it," how do you react when somebody tells you you did something good? How do you feel?

Neal: When they get done sayin' something nice, then you say "Thank you."

Dr. A.: That's right. That's a good answer. Did you know there are some people who have a hard time taking compliments? If somebody says something good to them, they have to say, "Oh no, that wasn't so good" or "So and so could have done better" or "Somebody else helped with it; that's why it's a good job," or they have to prove it's not good. They would say, "Oh, look here, look and see what's wrong with it." They run it down. They run themselves down. Why would anybody do that to themselves? Does anybody here do that to themselves? [A few nods; some parents smile understandingly.] Why do people have trouble taking compliments? [The children make no verbal response, but they look attentive.]

(*gently*) Maybe you guys didn't understand what I asked. (*thinking out loud*) There are some people who if you tell them you did a good job and you say, "Oh look what a nice job" or "I like the way your hair is fixed" or "That was a good hit you made," some people, if you say it to them, they'll really try to show you it wasn't good and show you what was wrong with it. What ideas do you have as to why somebody would run themselves down? It seems kind of funny doesn't it? Maybe you guys could ask your moms. [This teaches children to use parents as consultants.]

Mrs. P.: Neal, why is it that when somebody says something nice to you, you run yourself down?

Neal: (*smiles, looking embarrassed*)

Dr. A.: (*picking up nonverbal clue*) Because you're embarrassed?

Neal: I'm shy.

Dr. A.: Oh, some people get embarrassed and shy when somebody says something good about them. Part of growing up is being able to take compliments. The person who is complimenting really enjoys it. If your friend does something good and you say "Oh, congratulations," doesn't it make you feel good to give a compliment? [Kids nod.] Well, it would make the other person feel good to say, "Thanks, your opinion means a lot to me." Maybe some of the adults can give reasons why somebody would get embarrassed when they get a compliment.

Dr. E.: One reason could be that they're so used to getting yelled at that when somebody compliments them, they're so surprised. It's like a shock. Maybe they don't believe it, so their first reaction is to put themselves down since it has always been a habit. You know how easy it is to get into a habit and how difficult a bad habit is to break.

Dr. A.: Oh yes, I think I know what you're saying: that sometimes people get used to each other acting in certain ways, that it's kind of hard to change our attitudes, especially about people, either ourselves or somebody else. For example, if we know somebody who used to be clumsy in sports and then he started to try real hard and practice a lot of extra hours every day after school and soon he became one of the best in his class. At first it may be hard to think of him as a good athlete. We would have to adjust our thinking.

Dr. E.: Another reason why somebody may not like compliments is because he is afraid of what people might expect of him. If he does a real good job, then people may expect him to do it all the time like that.

Kurt: Yeah, like when you get an A on a spelling test, your mother thinks you should get it all the time.

Dr. A.: Well, if you could do it once, would you worry that you couldn't do it again?

Kurt: Well, nobody's perfect.

Dr. E.: That's right. We all have good days and bad days.

Several salient points from this session are worth mentioning. Techniques of behavior management that employ the use of exact numbers instead of vague generalizations will help both children and parents recognize improvements in behavior, however small the increment might be. In most instances, parents and children have a tendency to overlook improvement in behavior unless it is 100 percent.

This tendency could perpetuate a vicious cycle, especially when a child's sense of self-worth is conditioned on behaving perfectly. It is also important to note the method the therapist uses when direct questioning of the children elicits no response. In these instances, it is best for the therapist to elicit responses from the parents (or even other therapists present), using them as consultants. The parents' ability to point out good things about the child in public is a way to sweeten a previously intense negative relationship. Thus a triple benefit is the result: not only is the relationship promoted between parents and children, but the children's self-esteem is raised by hearing the positive comment, and the parent is taught a technique for nurturing and supporting the child.

8
You Don't Always Like
the One You Love

Love is a four-letter word that many mental health professionals eschew. Children, fortunately, are more realistic and brave (or foolhardy). They are usually willing to discuss love and its ramifications frankly, if only the adult introduces the topic.

Troubled children often crave love or signs of it and ineptly manipulate for it in ways that defeat their purpose, ways that result in further evidence to them of their fancied love deprivations. A few may even deliberately, though unconsciously (neurotically), sabotage their chances to experience love. Others may extract signs of love to such an irrational extent that they murder love.

One day the subject of love came up in a parents' group because one pair of parents was concerned about the lying their ten-year-old adopted son of four years, Tom, had become involved in. Not only was he lying, but he deliberately was not doing what he was supposed to do. When his parents caught him being good and reinforced him for the behavior by complimenting him, he would act babyish and talk baby talk. He would dress himself backward so they would have to dress him, and act immature. The parents, disgusted with him, would withdraw their approval. It seemed that one of the basic issues here was Tom's need for love and for reassurance that he was loved. After the children returned, Dr. A. introduced the discussion from the parents' group to the children:

Dr. A.: One of the things that the parents were talking about that's very important is love. They didn't really talk about it in those words but kind of talked around it. Who can tell me what love means?

Tom: It means that sombody cares about you.

Dr. A.: Why is love so important?

Tom: Well, everybody wants someone to care about him.

Dr. A.: Which is more important: to love or to have somebody to love you?

Bill: (*after some thought*) I think it's important to have somebody love you—but it's also important to have somebody to love also.

Vic: To have somebody love you.

Dr. A.: Tom, maybe you can explain to Vic [who is six years old] why it's important to have somebody to love also?

Tom: You have to be loved and have somebody to love. [Vic nods.]

Dr. A.: That's right. Happiness is based on being loved, being cared for by someone, and having someone that you can care for to give you some kind of meaning for doing things because it will make the other person happy. [Both Tom and Vic nod.] How can a person know he is loved? What are some ways people can show another that they love him?

Vic: People could give you things, like presents and toys and treats.

Dr. A.: Is there any other way?

Tom: They can do things with you.

Dr. A.: That's right! That is a good way of showing love. Are there any other ways? [No response.] Maybe there are some funny ways that love is shown, that don't look like love at first. [The children look puzzled.]

Tom: Well, they can tell you that they love you.

Dr. A.: How do you know that they mean it?

Tom: (*looking bewildered*)

Dr. A.: But what about some unusual ways of showing love? [The children still look puzzled.] OK, how about this. Suppose you love somebody, and they insist on walking out in the middle of a busy highway. It's dangerous, and they might get killed. What would you do about it?

Tom: I would tell him he should get out of the highway.

Dr. A.: What if he wouldn't?

Tom: I guess that would be up to him to decide.

Dr. A.: You mean you would let him get killed? What do you think, Andy? [Andy shrugs.] Let's think some more. Suppose this person was a lot younger, and he didn't know any better, and you knew he might get killed walking down the highway. What would you do about it? Would you make him get out of the highway?

Tom: I would tell him to get out of the highway. I would explain why he should.

Dr. A.: What if you had to hurt him to do it—like tie him up or drag him out of the highway. Would you do that? [After much thought, Tom reluctantly agreed that he would.] Vic, what about you? What would you do?

Vic: I wouldn't drag him out.

Dr. A.: [Dr. A. invites Tom to explain to Vic how it would be the right thing to do.] So to show that you really care about somebody, sometimes you have to do something that they might not really like, but it's really good for them in the long run. [The children nod.] What about punishment? Can punishment be a way somebody can show you they love you? A parent knows that a kid is doing something wrong that will get him in trouble or would make his friends turn against him—like if a kid punches their friends, maybe a parent should punish him. [The children look puzzled.] Is that a way of showing love?

Tom: I guess so.

Dr. A.: Is it good to have friends? Do you like to have friends? (*to Vic*) [Vic nods.] (*to Tom*) Is it good to have friends? [Tom nods.] And if your parents try to help you keep friends, is that showing you that they love you? [Both children nod.] If you're doing something like punching another kid, that makes him not want to be friends with you. Is it showing love if your parents try to get you to stop that? [Tom and Vic nod.] And if they punish you to make you stop, is that showing love? [Both nod.]

We've heard about a lot of different ways somebody shows they love you: if they say they love you, if they give you nice things, if they praise you, take care of you, or if they punish you in some way, stop you from doing things that may get you in trouble or lose friends—all kinds of different ways to know you're loved. Now suppose somebody gets hung up on just one way of knowing that they're loved. Maybe the only way they can feel loved is if they know they're being punished. What would you think of that?

Tom: Well, that's stupid. [He looks at Andy, who repeats Tom's remarks.]

Dr. A.: Well, I know some kids are just that way: that the only way they could be sure they're loved is if somebody was harassing them, punishing them, or doing something like that to them. They didn't seem to know any other way. What would you do in a case like that, if you had a friend like that who was always getting you to do something bad to him so he would know you cared about him?

Tom: I would tell him about the other ways he should know he's loved.

Dr. A.: Suppose he wouldn't believe you. He really couldn't get that idea through his head. What would you do? If somebody compliments him or praises him, he is not really sure about it. The only way he feels sure somebody loves him is if they do something nasty to him.

Tom: Well, I'd just explain to him. I'd make him understand.

Dr. A.: But suppose he didn't understand, no matter what you did.

Tom: Well, I guess I'd just be stuck. I wouldn't know what to do. [He looks really perplexed.]

Dr. A.: Yeah, you know I think parents really get into that fix; parents don't know how they can get their kids to understand they're loved in other ways.

Toms' mother: That's just the way I feel. [Tom looks surprised, and then turns to his mother with apparently increased understanding and then lapses into sheepish pensiveness.]

Sometimes children bring up the topic of love themselves. Dr. A. had been attempting a transition from a discussion on teamwork in the children's group to the topic of rewards that the parents had been concerned about in their group. He had just made the point that teamwork is important in families, and one way for families to work together is to reward each other.

Doug: And love each other!

Dr. A.:   Love each other? Should a family love each other? What do the rest of you think? [Most children nod.] Bob? Ned? [Both nod.] OK. Everybody agrees that in a family, everybody should love each other. What does love mean?

Eugene: Caring about each other.

Dr. A.:   Very good.

Doug: Worrying about each other.

Dr. A.:   That's very good because a lot of kids wouldn't think about worrying about each other. Parents do, though. They do a lot of worrying because they love you. I'm glad no one said that love means that you like each other. Usually you like the person you love and love the person you like. What is the difference between liking and loving? You already said loving was worrying and caring about the person.

Theresa: They're a little bit alike, but loving is more.

Dr. A.:   Would you believe that you could love somebody and not like them? How do you think that could be? I see some of the grown-ups nodding their heads.

Mrs. X.:   You could love somebody and not like them. You can have deep feelings but not like what they do or how they act or the way they talk.

Dr. A.:   Love is caring and worrying about somebody. Love is an action, something you do. A commitment from somebody. If they really love you, you can count on them to stick by you no matter what happens. But liking is enjoying being with someone; it's fun to be with them. It's great to both like and love somebody. Which is more important?

Theresa: To love.

9
Rewards

Principles of behavior modification are used and taught throughout all segments of multifamily sandwich group therapy as part of the multimodal approach. These principles will not be reviewed here in any systematic way but are integrated into many chapters throughout the book, just as they are integrated throughout the group. For example, chapter 4 includes an explanation of the reward hierarchy as an example of a mini-lecture. The following transcript illustrates another common need for clarification about rewards. It starts in the middle of the parents' group and runs over into the last parent-child segment.

Mrs. X.: With Ned, he always says, "What are you going to give me if I do this?" I say, "What are you going to give me if I give you your dinner tonight and do this and this and this that I don't particularly want to do? I don't want to get up and go to work in the morning but I am going to get up, and you're going to go to school in the morning." We do use the reward system to a certain extent, but, it's not a bribery-type thing.

Mrs. Y.: (*angrily*)Well, I like to be the one to reward. I don't want Bob to be the one to say to me, "I'll do this and this, if you give me this or pay me a dollar." I want to be the one to give the reward [Mrs. X. is nodding.] and say, "you know, you were such a good boy you can have an extra half-hour of television before bedtime" or "You can earn an extra fifteen cents of an allowance." I tell him that if he listens or does what he is told, then I continue it. I tell him if he would listen, then he wouldn't have to be yelled at, at home, and he wouldn't have to have all these restrictions. I talk to him like an adult.

It is tempting here to explore Mrs. Y.'s misguided efforts to reason with her son, which undoubtedly come across as nagging and may set expectations beyond his present capacity. This could make a productive topic, but at this time it would distract from a theme that seems better established, with two parents already stating their concern.

Dr. A.: You've raised a very important point, and that's the distinction among bribery, contract, and reward. I think you are quite right in saying that you need to be the one to decide on the reward. Parents need to be in control of that. It's the whole idea of behavior modification that the behavior manager controls the rewards; you control the goods. It necessitates sometimes putting a lock on the cupboard if the reward is a cookie (if you do not want him to get into the cookie jar on his own). If it's to stay up late to watch a special television show to reward him for something he's done, then you have to make sure he doesn't sneak and watch it anyway when he hasn't earned the reward.

You also have to make sure he's not getting a greater reward by not doing what he is supposed to do. Maybe it's more rewarding to him to have you fussing and yelling at him for not doing it than the reward would be.

Now, what's the difference between a bribe and a reward? One difference is that a bribe is for doing something wrong. Another is that a bribe often is given before the fact. For example, you are a highway contractor and you go to a highway official and you say, "Here's half of a $1,000 bill, and you get the other half after I'm awarded the contract." A reward is given after the fact. You do your job and collect your paycheck. I don't think anyone of us would consider our hard-earned paycheck bribery. Likewise, a kid does his chores, and then he gets a privilege. He doesn't get the privilege before he does his chores. So a reward comes afterward, for doing something good; a bribe comes before for something bad.

Another distinction is a bonus and a contract. A bonus is something that is freely given; it is one kind of reward. The other kind of reward is to contract for a reward, like a paycheck. In a sense, the paycheck is a reward for working. Bribery is in a sense a contract, but an illegal, immoral contract. [During this explanation, the children have come back from their separate group.]

You kids probably noticed that we were talking about rewards and goodies and things like that. First, why don't you kids tell us what you did in your separate group. [Dr. A. looks around the room, and Doug is the first to raise his hand.] OK, Doug, why don't you tell us what you did.

Doug: We played kickball and won. [This is an unusual privilege because competitive activities are usually deemphasized.]

Dr. A.: How do you play kickball?

Vance: Someone throws the ball to you, you kick it, and then you run.

Dr. A.: Do all the adults understand from Vance's description? [The adults nod.] Good. That's an important skill, to be able to tell about something and have somebody understand. What is the value of playing kickball?

Vance: It's like baseball.

Dr. A.: OK, so you can learn how to play baseball from playing kickball. Anything else? Another thing that you said, Doug, is that your team won. What does a team mean? Does a team mean just doing whatever you want to do? Is each person trying to do their own thing?

Doug: No.

Dr. A.: OK. Teamwork is important to learn. One of the places that you have teamwork is between you and your parents, or you should have. In some families, the parents and kids are not working together as a team, and that causes problems and everybody loses. A team that doesn't work together is a team that is not going to win. Right? [The children nod.] One of the things we need to talk about here is how your family can become a winning team. One of the ways, one of the things the parents were talking about, is rewards. One way to keep a family working together well is to reward each other. [Doug looks as if he has something pressing to share.] Doug, what is it?

Doug: And love each other!

Dr. A. had several options in response to Doug's tangential comments: Ignore it; question its relevance; ask for clarification; explore it in reference to the agenda topic; reinterpret or reframe it as a valuable relevant comment; or treat it as an expansion of the agenda topic and then tie it back in.

Dr. A.: Love each other? Should a family love each other? What do the rest of you think? [Most children nod.] Bob? Ned? [Both nod.] OK. Everybody agrees that in a family everybody should love each other. What does love mean?

Here a section of interaction has been deleted and moved to chapter 8.

Dr. A. followed the love tangent suggested by Doug for a few minutes before tying it back in like this:

Dr. A.:   I think that what happens in some of your families is that you love each other, but you find it very hard to like each other because of the things you kids do. Is that right? [Group nods.] One of the things we need to do is find ways to like each other. One of the things your parents were talking about that they would like to be able to do is to give you rewards for doing good things. Who can tell me what a reward is? [Hands up.] Ned, what is it?

Ned: It is when I memorize my tables, I get to stay up. But I don't get many rewards.

Dr. A.:   So this is a reward your mother and you agreed on ahead of time. That's good. But what if a kid says, "You owe me $15 because I did such and such," and there really wasn't any agreement ahead of time? What would you think of that? [The children look thoughtful.] What if Mom says, "I'm short of money; I can't afford it this week"? What do you think of that?

Ned: I did that to my mother.

Dr. A.:   Well, who do you think is in charge of whether you get something like that? [Bob's hand goes up.] Bob?

Bob: (*points to Mom*) [Group applauds.]

The following transcript is a complete discussion section from the last segment of a group. During this section, the children usually discuss a topic from the separate parents' group recalled by the group leader; only occasional comments are inserted by parents. This particular session was unusual in being dominated by the adults, possibly because of the great feeling among some parents about the topic. During the parents' group, there had been much complaint about the children's behavior being worse in the summer and about their loss of interest in projects or slacking to trivial projects.

Dr. M.:   One of the things that came up in the parents' group is the question, "Why do kids behave worse in the summer?" [The children look puzzled.]

Dr. A.:   Are big people allowed to answer? I have an idea. I think after a while, maybe kids feel like they need a vacation. We have summer vacation from school, and maybe some kids think they should have a summer vacation from behaving, too.

Deanna: If you're good and act good all the time, then you don't have to come here.

Dr. M.: Very good. Any others?

Mr. F.: I wonder if in our situation, where both parents work and they're only home on the weekends, that's harder, because on vacation you don't have that structure of going to the sitter and doing things at certain times. You kind of forget about the structured part of your goal because you're more relaxed. You might get to stay up later, and you kind of forget about those things.

Dr. A.: Forgetting can be OK sometimes after the pressing problem is taken care of. Maybe there's a real crisis or problem, and everybody gets organized to do something about it and then it works, so you don't need to worry so much about it anymore; things are going better, so people don't see any great need. We don't use these techniques of counting, keeping track, stars, and rewards unless it is something that's really bothering us. It's human nature to let up after a while. You put an effort into something, you make an improvement, and you want to sit back and enjoy what you've accomplished.

Dr. M.: Another thing—maybe kids pick a project that's not really important to them; maybe they just pick something because they think it's going to be easy, or they pick something they think their mother or father wants them to pick, but they don't see any need for it or don't see why it's important. Then what's the point of doing it?

Mrs. C.: But they may not realize what's important to begin with, and you can't just let them pick what they want.

Dr. A.: Why not?

Mrs. C.: They keep avoiding the problem. They know they're doing wrong but if you don't make them do it, they'll just keep avoiding the problem.

Dr. A.: You're assuming the project has to be one the parent considers important.

Mrs. C.:   Not all the time, but they shouldn't avoid really important issues.

Dr. A.:   I agree that that could be a danger, too. If the kid is avoiding important things, that is something that shouldn't be allowed to continue forever, but I think it's all right for a kid once in a while to pick something that's important to him even if it's not to you, like, for example, to make a new friend. Maybe that's not important to the parents. They think he has plenty of friends already—but maybe to him, he feels like he really doesn't have enough friends. So he wants to make a new friend. I don't see anything wrong with taking that for a project. But if he avoids and never takes for a project something that the parents agree is a problem, then I agree that's bad, too. Could you give an example of something you think a kid should not take for a project? [There is no response from Mrs. C.] Anybody?

Mrs. C.:   I can't think of anything, but maybe they shouldn't keep picking the same thing.

Dr. A.:   OK. [Dr. A. finally perceives that what the parents are really complaining about is feeling helpless, at the mercy of the child's whim about the project.] I just had an idea. What if the parents pick a project that they think is important, to get the kid to work on a certain thing that they think is important and the kid doesn't?

Mrs. F.:   For the project to work, you have to have willingness on the part of the child. They have to want to change.

Dr. A.:   Not necessarily. I think it's possible for parents to pick a project where they want to change something about the kid's behavior. The kid may not be interested in it, but I think you can devise a plan that will accomplish it. For example, maybe you want to get him to quit tracking mud into the house. He really couldn't care less. He realizes that humans and pigs have common physiology, and thinks they ought to behave the same way [laughter from group], but it's important to you to keep him from tracking mud in. So you set up a behavior modification paradigm whereby he gets rewarded for taking his muddy boots off at the door. Now, if he takes them off at the door, he can't be tracking mud in. The two things are incompatible. And all you have to do is find the right reinforcer, and you can gradually shape his behavior for taking his boots off at the door—even though he wasn't interested at all in doing that in the first place.

Mrs. G.: About picking an easier project instead of a difficult one, is it possible that sometimes if a child picks that type of goal that he doesn't feel confident? Maybe you should let him for a period of time pick an easier goal that he can have success with and maybe later he can pick a harder goal. [Note how constructively and understandingly the parents respond after Dr. A. showed them how they could have some control and power.]

Dr. A.: That's a very good point. Did everybody else understand that? Pick something you can do, then do it, get that under your belt; and then you get a little stronger. Then you have the motivation to tackle something bigger and gradually work up the line. Maybe you don't necessarily want to start with the most important item, but start with the thing you can do and work gradually to harder things. That might make more sense than trying to start with the most important things, which might be too hard to do until you have had practice doing easier things.

Mrs. C.: But even the smallest goals to one certain child might be the hardest to another. So if you're making an attempt and really trying, that is the accomplishment.

Dr. A.: You said something very important and that is, to you the effort is important. I want to make sure the kids all hear that. Most parents feel the same way. If you can see that your kid is trying, that counts for something. Maybe he doesn't succeed every time, but he's trying, and you know that eventually he's going to succeed if he keeps trying.

Mrs. D.: If there is even the least little bit of cooperation, then it has to be recognized, whether there is reprimand or not. Even small things are an issue.

Dr. A.: The other thing you said that is important is that what is easy for one kid may be hard for another. Now, we saw a good example of that today down in the gym because some kids had trouble jumping rope and other kids found that easy. But maybe somebody who could jump a rope easily had trouble crawling through the inner tube. Or somebody who had found both of those easy had trouble on the scooter board. So each person has certain things they're good at and other things they're not so good at, and they can improve both of those. You have a different standard for different jobs. If it's hard for them, then a little bit of success is an improvement. If it's easy for them, then you expect more in that area.

Mrs. B.: There are limitations that they have. If they want to improve on them, the thought and the willingness to try are important, and we should recognize even little improvements.

Dr. A.: I think what you're talking about now is feedback; you let them know how they're doing. And I guess that makes a good transition to the formal feedback that we provide here: the star charts.

10
Planning, Structure, Organization, Control, Self-Control, and the Art of Umpire Acceptance

Planning, self-structuring, and cooperating with the structure provided by others are some of the ways people can get organized and develop self-control. In this vignette Dr. A. was attempting to help the children understand and organize their behavior by reviewing the importance of planning:

Dr. A.: In order to be a good student or athlete, you have to listen, remember, and then what?

Children: Do it!

Dr. A.: How do you know the right thing to do? What is between hearing and doing? [The children look puzzled.] Well, you can use your ears for hearing and your hands, feet, and eyes in coordinating it, but what comes in between when you listen to what someone tells you and when you do it?

Kurt: You're using your brain.

Dr. A.: Right, you're using your brain to do what? [The children look puzzled.] If you listen and do it without thinking about it, you could get into trouble. There is a step in between that helps you do a better job or saves you from making a mistake. You do it every week on your projects, and if you don't do it, you have problems.

Kurt and
Tom: (*smiling in unison*) We plan!

Dr. A.: Right. Planning is going through it in your head before you actually do it with your feet. It's taking action in your brain to think it out ahead of time, to make sure you're going to do it right.

Note the Socratic questioning, with the provision of more and more hints until the children guessed the answer. Sometimes, though, the children do not give the expected answer. They may even seem counterproductive. In the following vignette, Andy seemed to disprove the importance of planning (after first attempting the forgetting role). Dr. A.'s clinical curiosity turned a discouraging report into a therapeutic opportunity. Dr. A. had just asked Andy to report on his project.

Andy   I forgot my assignment.

Dr. A.:   Maybe somebody here can help you remember. Maybe your mother can give you a hint.

Andy: Oh, going to bed on time.

Dr. A.:   Going to bed on time was your goal. That's right. Now what was your plan? Each time you have a goal and to get to the goal, you need _____.

Andy: (*interrupting*) I forgot my plan.

Dr. A.:   Oh. (*pause*) Did you go to bed on time?

Andy: Yeah. [Dr. A. looks at mom for confirmation.]

Andy's
mother: He went to bed on time sometimes.

Dr. A.:   Was it an improvement over last week? [Andy's mother nods.] That's interesting. How do you suppose that can be? Andy says he forgot his assignment, but he ended up doing it anyway. He was going to go to bed on time, and the way he was going to remember was to have some fun before he went to bed; that would kind of be like an incentive to hurry up and get ready for bed. Now his mother said he improved, and Andy said he forgot his plan. How do you suppose that can be? How can you forget what you're supposed to do and still go ahead and do it? Did that happen to any of you? Kurt? Charles? [The children look puzzled but receptive. This is a good time to program them with constructive suggestions.]
          You know, sometimes we have a way of doing things without

thinking about them. If we get things organized in our mind, then we don't have to think about it all the time. And that's one of the things you're working on in here: to get in the habit of getting organized so you can do things right without thinking. If you get in the habit of sitting still, paying attention, walking down the hall without bothering anyone, and finishing up things, then you won't have to think about it anymore. It is just like someone learning how to drive; once they learn to do it, they don't have to think about it anymore. So you succeeded a little bit, Andy. Can you nail it down to how many times it was? Then I'll ask your mother, to check how close your guess is. [Andy grins with pleasure.] This is important, learning to observe your own behavior.

Control

In another session, Dr. A. was explaining behavior to the children with the implicit message, "If you cannot control your behavior, your parents need to help you."

Dr. A.:   (*to the children*) Have you heard of the word *control*? What does control mean?

Craig: There are two kinds. One is like you have with a car. One is like control with a helicopter, and one is like controlling the body.

Dr. A.:   I'm glad you answered the question in three ways because there are several types of control, such as controlling emotions, behavior, or temper, so you don't have a tantrum. What kinds of control are there? Kurt? Tom? Vic? What are the meanings? You control your body, but what else can you control?

Bob: You can control your feelings.

Craig's   You can control another person. [She and Craig have been battling
mother: over control for some time now.]

Dr. A.:   Control another person! How much can you control another person?

Craig: I feel like a slave. (*mimicking his mother*) "Do this, do that . . ."
[He becomes annoying by continuing to mimic his mother with no sign of stopping.]

Dr. A.:   (*to Craig*) Can you control your mouth?

Craig: No. [He continues mouthing off, and Dr. A. turns to other children.]

Dr. A.:   Do the other kids like to be in control?

Sarah: I like it a little.

Dr. A.:   What about you, Kurt?

Kurt: Yes. [He can hardly be heard because of Craig's loud interruptions.]

Dr. A.:   Craig, right now I'd like you to control your mouth.

Craig: If it's over three minutes, forget it!

Craig has issued a challenge that could easily turn into a useless or even destructive power struggle, similar to those reported by Craig's mother to occur between her and Craig at home. It was essential for the group leader to model for Craig's mother a method for dealing with such challenges in a way other than being hooked into a shouting match or argument at the child's level—an "I can make you do it" trap. One option could have been to give the child time-out to cool off in a supportive, nonpunitive way, such as, "Craig, I can understand how hard it is for you to be quiet, but it would not be fair to the other kids if I let you do all the talking. So I'm going to let you go back to the observation room where you can see and hear what is going on but cannot interrupt. As soon as you can get your mouth under control [note the implication that it is something he wants to do and eventually will be able to do], you can return to the group."

A better option when possible is to find the silver lining in the child's challenge and respond to that, ignoring the hostile elements. Craig's announcement that he could not do it longer than three minutes was an implicit invitation to be required to do it for three minutes. Dr. A. chose to attend to this positive implication of what overtly sounded negative. The good results that followed are typical of what can be acomplished by ferreting out and attending to the positive aspects of a hostile child's negative-sounding communications.

Craig: If it's over three minutes, forget it!

Dr. A.: OK, let's try it for three minutes. Can you practice some self-control right now? [Under his breath, Craig sarcastically mutters, "The slave will agree to it."]

Dr. A.: (*to the rest of the group*) OK, now: can you absolutely control another person?

Group: No!

Dr. A.: What about in a family? Can you control other family members?

Kurt: Yes.

Dr. A.: Well, I guess we all agree in a family some people can get others to do things they want. Who in your family can get you to do what they want?

Tom: My mother and father.

Dr. A.: Can they really?

Tom: Sometimes. [This discussion continues a few more minutes, resulting in the realization that although parents can exert of lot of influence on children, the children are responsible for self-control.]

Dr. A.: OK, Craig. Time's up. That was excellent self-control. You can do it if you really concentrate and plan what you're going to do, and as long as you take it in small steps, a few minutes at a time. [Craig's attitude the rest of this group and in subsequent groups was cooperative and constructive.]

Antidote for Accidents

Many children are accident prone for a variety of reasons: neurological incoordination, impulsiveness, high activity level, poor ability to learn from experience, tendency to get into things, and failure to plan ahead. Consequently their parents worry about their vulnerability in ways that the child may consider overcontrol or nagging.

Dr. A.: (*to children*) Something came up during the parents' group that I thought you kids would be interested in. The parents were concerned about you kids having accidents! Why do you think your parents would worry about you kids having accidents? [The children look puzzled.] Well, do you think it's just because its a big nuisance and expense, and they don't want to have to bother with that?

Ned: They don't want you to hurt yourself, cuz it hurts.

Dr. A.: You mean they don't want you to be in pain. Is that it?

Ned: Yeah, cuz they care for you.

Dr. A.: Because they care for you; that's right. They don't want you to have an accident, because if you have an accident, then you'll be in pain, and they love you and don't want you to be hurting. How come you have so many accidents? What causes accidents? [Donna's had goes up.] Donna?

Donna: Cuz you don't look where you are going.

Dr. A.: OK, Ned, anything else?

Ned: You don't pay any attention to what you're doing, so you end up bumping into something.

Dr. A.: I guess you two agree that you have an accident when you don't look what you're doing or don't pay attention to where you're going. OK, what else?

Ned: If you're careless.

Dr. A.: What does *careless* mean?

Ned: If you're doing something and then something else happens and you didn't know about it!

Dr. A.: You mean if you don't think ahead, then you're careless. How does thinking ahead help you keep from having an accident? [Doug's hand goes up.] Doug?

Doug: If you don't think ahead, you get into trouble.

Dr. A.: Oh, thinking ahead or planning, where you go through it in your mind, that can keep you from having an accident, can't it? Maybe you can prevent accidents by thinking ahead to other people, too, like what it'll do to the other guy.

Umpiring

In the parents' group the first week of summer vacation, there had been complaints that the children seemed to cast aside all discipline when school closed. They began ignoring chores and home rules and did not even report where they were going.

When the children returned from their activities, they complained that they had not been able to enjoy a wiffle ball game because of arguments in the absence of an umpire. Ordinarily competitive activities are discouraged in the children's group, but this day the six children persuaded the occupational therapist that they all needed practice in teamwork, cooperation, and avoiding arguments; they were right.

Aaron: "Argue-ball" is no fun. [Laughter from group.]

Vince: We should have had an umpire or referee.

Dr. A.: Do the rest of you agree that an umpire would be good? [All children nod or say "yes."] What for? What good is an umpire? [Walt's hand goes up.] Walt?

Walt: So we can get the job done.

Aaron: We could have fun instead of arguing.

Dr. A.: So an umpire helps keep things going in an orderly way so you can have more fun. Do you all agree? [The children nod.] Tell me: Who's the umpire for the summer? [The children look puzzled.] Who's the umpire at home?

Several
children: *(with "aha!" smile)* Oh! [Hands up.]

Mike: Mom!

Dr. A.: Right! Your parents are the umpires and referees at home, and teachers are at school. In the summer you need to do what the home umpires say to have a fun summer.

Note that the transition has been made from segment 1 of the last slice (children's report of their activities) to segment 2 (topic from parents' group). It would have been desirable for Dr. A. to insert a comment like, "That brings us to something your parents were talking about in their group."

Dr. A.:   Why should you do what mom or dad says? [Dr. A. asked a question for which he had just given the answer. This technique reinforces attentiveness, with an immediate opportunity for successful recitation.]

Kim: If we behave, we'll stay out of trouble.

Dr. A.:   Right. Are there any other reasons for behaving?

Aaron: They'll let you go to a friend's house on your bike. [He goes into an elaborate description of how to earn more freedom.]

Dr. A.:   It sounds like another reason for behaving is that you can get more privileges and freedom if you behave. If you behave well, they'll let you ride your bike, let you visit somebody.

Aaron: If they give you a time to come home on time, like, say, 3:30, and you come home at 3:30, well, they might let you go out from 3:30 to 5:30.

Dr. A.:   OK. Did the rest of you understand that? Another reason for behaving is that you get more things if you handle the first one well. [Group nods.] What else?

Vince: My daddy always told me about the camper. He said if I keep it clean and take responsibility, I'll have it someday—like I'll clean up a lot, I'll sweep inside, and keep it clean—and "it'll be nice when you get it."

Dr. A.:   That brings up something important. One reason for behaving is that it is good practice for when you grow up. If you behave by yourself when you are a kid, it is easy when you grow up.

Aaron: Well, I don't behave all the time; sometimes I do, and I like it better then. If you behave and stay out of trouble now, then you're better than if you start getting in big trouble in high school.

Dr. A.:   So you've given two more reasons now, Aaron. It makes you feel good to behave good. It's nice to be a good person, and you feel good inside when you behave well. It's like success: you know you can do it. The other thing is that it is going to be harder to behave in high school than now, so if you don't practice it now, you'll really get in trouble then. Any other reasons? [No response.] You've come up with some really good ones. The one I like best is the one about feeling good. How many have had that? You feel good when you behave well. [Several nod.] How about you, Konrad?

Konrad: Yes.

Dr. A.:   [Three-year-old Dave puts up hand and points to self.] You too, Dave? [Dave nods and grins.] I think that is one of the best reasons. That is the reason to behave: because it makes you feel good to behave. That's part of growing up.

11
Power Struggles

S ome children are locked into an oppositional or passive-aggressive power struggle with their parents. Most such parents welcome advice on how to break up the power struggle and promote a more supportive and enjoyable relationship with the child. A few parents, however, seem to relish the struggle, either because they like the tragic hero or martyr role or because they unconsciously want an excuse to reject the child.

"Mary, Mary, Quite Contrary, How Does Your Mother Blow?"

The following transcript documents Dr. A.'s struggles to manage a rejecting, angry, help-rejecting hypomanic mother in the parents' group. It is of interest not only because it is rich in parental psychopathology but also because the reader can enjoy listing ways that Dr. A. could have been more effective, efficient, therapeutic, or professional. Before concluding that this mother should be dropped from the group in favor of individual help, notice that the most useful interventions seemed to issue from other parents in the group.

This transcript is unusual in the amount of confronting and challenging that Dr. A. felt obliged to pursue with Mrs. Z. With most parents (and most parents' groups), a more supportive, consultative, or facilitative role can be assumed.

Mrs. Z.: (*talking about daughter Mary's oppositional behavior*) She won't do anything. For mealtime I feel like I should make a tape recording that says, "Don't eat your food." [Laughter from the other six parents in the group.]

Dr. A.: What would happen if you didn't tell Mary to eat her food?

Mrs. Z.:   She has sat at the table for two hours with a plate of cold soup, twisting her hair. Last night I had to wash her hair because she gets food in it from twisting it. I said to her, "Why do you do this? Why do you twist your hair?" "I have to be doing something with my fingers; I have to do something with my fingers." I can't stand it. You try to hold her hands to stop her from doing it, and she just gets horrible.

Dr. A.:   Does anyone have any ideas about handling this? [The parents look puzzled.] What would happen if you wouldn't make her eat?

Mrs. Z.:   She wouldn't eat then. She won't.

Dr. A.:   Forever? She'll just starve to death?

Mrs. Z.:   Exactly. [Score one for Mrs. Z. Dr. A.'s attempted reductio ad absurdum is stymied. Mrs. B. comes to the rescue.]

Mrs. B.:   That was a big problem I went through, and Dr. S. suggested to me that to relieve the tension of this, I should offer the food and if she doesn't eat it, then take it away. There still are some foods my son won't eat, but I don't push him.

Mrs. Z.:   I look in her lunch box from school, and I see she only takes one bite out of her sandwich. If I look into her thermos, I see it's the same amount. I ask her, "How can you go the entire day without drinking? Don't you get thirsty?"

Mr. B.:   Dr. A. once told us that having a balanced breakfast is good. We try to have a better balanced meal in the morning, but still he doesn't always eat it.

Dr. A.:   (*to Mr. and Mrs. B.*) Some of his loss of appetite is from the side effects of medicine.

Dr. A. had two reasons for this apparently irrelevant comment. He wished to remind the parents subtly that the child may not be at fault in not eating or not doing other things; there may be reasonable causes or explanations. Second, Mrs. Z. had been pushing for inappropriate medication for her daughter, and he wished to point out that medicine might well make one of the things worse that Mrs. Z. is complaining about.

Mrs. Z.:   Mary will do these ridiculous things. She'll cough and cough and cough until she starts gagging and wretching. We send her away from the table and say, "Go to the bathroom or go to your bedroom until you stop coughing; then you can come back to the table." My mother comes to visit us, and she drives my mother crazy, too. My mother stands on her head trying to get this kid to eat. Today is the first day since we've been here a week ago that she's in a pleasant mood. I tried your blanket wrap, and I think if she had the power to kill me, she would. [Laughter from the group.]

Dr. A.: Was this at a time when she was agitated or when she was just having trouble getting to sleep?

Mrs. Z.: I tried it several times; she just became increasingly more angry. She has been so hostile this week . . . [Now Mrs. Z. switches to complaining about her one-year-old daughter, Dana, without bothering to specify.] Yesterday, she screamed from 4:00 in the morning until I finally got her to sleep that evening at 8:30. Just screaming and screaming, like someone was killing her—no tears. I had a migraine and was ready to go berserk. Then I put her bottle on the walker after she got up. She hurled it; water was everywhere. I gave her a toy, and she threw it across the room.

[Mrs. Z. has become increasingly theatrical and is obviously entertaining the other parents. Dr. A. decides that problem solving cannot proceed until the theatrics-entertainment-reinforcing-attention cycle is exposed and discredited.]

Dr. A.: (*to Mrs. Z.*) You know, you're being cheated. Erma Bombeck makes a million dollars for this kind of stuff. [Laughter from the rest of the group.] [Dr. A. could be criticized for unnecessary use of hostility in this succinct metaphorical interpretation but even in retrospect expresses no remorse.]

Mrs. Z.: (*slightly subdued*) To me it's not funny. Yesterday she kept hitting herself, like she's just so angry. There is nothing you can do.

Dr. A.: What would your next move be? Essentially, I guess I hear you saying that she's hopeless and you can't do anything with her, that you tried everything; different ideas other people have given you, different ideas of your own, and nothing has worked.

Mrs. Z.: Nothing has worked.

Dr. A.:   Well, what do you want to do? Where do you want to go from here?

Mrs. Z.: I don't know. That's why I'm here. I'm waiting for you to tell me. I'm waiting. I keep thinking baby must be having some bad headaches. That she has to be in terrific pain because of the way she screams and hits herself in the head. She'll be in a fabulous mood, and then as if you pushed a button, she'll switch and scream and scream for two and three hours. I've slept in her room for two weeks to observe what she does.

Dr. A.:   Are you talking about Dana?

Mrs. Z.: Yes.

Dr. A.:   OK, I thought you were talking about Mary. When did you switch from talking about Mary to talking about Dana?

Mrs. Z.: Yesterday was the worst day I have ever had. [Good try, Mrs. Z., but Dr. A. is not shaken off so easily.]

Dr. A.:   I get the feeling that this is similar: that what Mary has put you through, Dana is putting you through, too. Does anyone else have this experience of the younger child kind of following along what the older one has done? [All the parents nod in agreement.]

Mrs. C.: I figure it must be me. There must be something I'm doing that's causing this. [Dr. A. failed to capitalize on Mrs. C.'s gem as he should have in this context. He was sidetracked by a reflex attempt to empathize and assuage Mrs. C.'s unproductive guilt. This reflex is therapeutic in most instances but was second best here.]

Dr. A.:   Are you blaming yourself?

Mrs. C.: I just don't understand this. I never treated my mother like this.

Mrs. Z.: I don't understand, either. Mary has everything she could possibly want. She goes to expensive private schools; we have done without just about everything to give her; like expensive handmade wooden toys, expensive dolls, tons of books, etc. Going anywhere with them is a nightmare.

Dr. A.:   Has anyone else had this experience?

Mrs. C.: Yeah, it seems as if the more you give them, the worse they get. I'm at a point now where I've been bringing him here, and he gets worse. You're investing all this time, energy, and money into the child and they're getting worse. When is this ever gonna get better? Where is the hope? Give us some.

Mrs. D.: We've been coming here for a couple of weeks now. I really think my son has finally got the message. He listens to me now. With Dana, I really empathize with you. We went through the very same thing with my older one. [Note that Mrs. D. has effectively responded to the request for hope that Mrs. C. directed to Dr. A.]

Mrs. Z.: Well, I just figured that there had to be something wrong physically. We have gone to numerous doctors. We found out that she does have many problems: allergies, deformed hip socket. But neurologically she was OK, and it was finally the neurologist, Dr. B., who recommended us to you. We can't even go to anyone's house with the kids. They request us to get a babysitter. No one will come to our house.

Dr. A.: How does the teacher handle all this at school?

Mrs. Z.: Mary is fabulous at school.

Dr. A.: So what has the teacher shared with you about handling her? Maybe you can use some of her ideas at home.

Mrs. Z.: I've had conferences and conferences with her. She just doesn't understand what's wrong with Mary at home. They would say Mary is a wonderful student: she minds, she listens to directions and does her work. They could not understand.

Dr. A.: Have you tried observing her in the classroom?

Mrs. Z.: Yes.

Dr. A.: How'd she do?

Mrs. Z.: She behaved beautifully except for twisting her hair in knots.

Dr. A.: The teacher doesn't mind her twisting her hair in knots?

Mrs. Z.: They found that if they ignore it, she would stop doing it.

Dr. A.:   Did she stop?

Mrs. Z.:   No. I threaten her all the time, that I'm gonna cut it off.

Dr. A.:   Is she doing any harm to it?

Mrs. Z.:   Oh, yes. You should see her ends. Beauticians say it is damaged.

Mrs. B.:   Although my problems were not quite like yours, I found out that I had to admit that I was a problem to my son; that he was a problem to me. I told him that he was a problem to me, and I had to get help for us. I've been coming here for five weeks, and things have gotten better already. I've found out how to cope better. I couldn't give him affection when he got on my nerves so bad. I started doing things with him now since he's doing better; I tell him he's earned it.

Dr. A.:   Have you required that of Mary? That she earn things?

Mrs. Z.:   Yes, but you know she put my mother in the hospital?

Dr. A.:   Can you stand to hear some good news?

Mrs. Z.:   (*sheepishly*) Yes.

Dr. A.:   Can you see one silver lining in the whole thing? She behaves well at school but like hell at home. I'm wondering how many parents would be willing to trade with you? They can handle their child at home, but they can't get him to behave at school. [Four of the six other parents nod knowingly.]

Mrs. C.:   Yeah, they call home every other week. He's not allowed to go to gym or music, etc. He gets in trouble on the bus all the time.

Mrs. Z. appears thoughtful. Her destructive criticism of her daughters, which she also had been indulging in in their presence, became less strident in the remainder of this session and the following week.

This parents' group was unusual in the extent to which Mrs. Z. dominated it. Even Dr. A. was hooked into focusing on her. To some extent, it was necessary to challenge her, but on at least one occasion he returned the floor to her after Mrs. B. had effectively taken it (the earning interchange). Ordinarily each parent who had not verbalized spontaneously halfway through the group would have been invited to comment. The three nonverbal parents (out of seven present) participated by smiles, nods, laughter, grimaces, groans, gestures, and attentional focus and generally supported Mrs. B., Mrs. C., and Mrs. D. Invitations for them to verbalize their opinions and feelings may have elicited a broader counterbalance to Mrs. Z. and allowed Dr. A. to switch more from the role of challenger to the role of facilitator.

Parent Power

Some parents have the opposite problem from Mrs. Z.: instead of overdirecting and overreacting, they capitulate and fail to react enough to set reasonable limits on a violent child who seems out of control. They need to be taught methods of controlling the child when needed. The holding techniques advocated by Friedman and associates[1] and by Henderson and associates[2] can be demonstrated right in the group. In some cases it seems best to have a staff member hold the child the first time to show the parent it works, but in many cases the parent can be coached right from the beginning to do it in the group with the support of other parents and staff.

The holding involves any of several noninjurious restraints of the child. One example is for the child to be facing away from the adult with arms crossed, held by the wrists in a sitting position so that biting, scratching, and kicking are impossible. The important thing is for neither the adult nor child to be hurt. However long it takes, the restraint is not relaxed until the child calms and agrees not to restart the unacceptable behavior.

Such a resort is seldom necessary; most hyperactivity can be calmed by the techniques described in chapter 3, including the blanket roll. But an occasional violent child may need such restraint, and it should not be avoided out of embarrassment. The parents will take their cue from the professionals regarding the hopelessness or feasibility and necessity of limiting the child's aggression.

Notes

1. R. Friedman, K. Dreizen, et al, "Parent power: A holding technique in the treatment of omnipotent children," *Int. J. Fam. Counsel.* 6 (1978):66–73.

2. A. Henderson, I. Dahlin, C. Partridge, et al, "A hypothesis on the etiology of hyperactivity, with a pilot study report of related non drug therapy," *Pediatrics, 52* (1973):4.

12
Competition and Fairness

C ompetition, excessive competitiveness, and cheating in the service of competition are common problems whenever children are compared to each other on some standard or when win-lose games are played. Winning and losing are downplayed in the activities provided for the children's group, and many of the activities do not have winners and losers. Nevertheless, competitiveness, cheating, and complaints of unfairness often crop up, providing grit for the therapeutic mill of the last segment of group.

Behavior- and learning-disordered children are more vulnerable than most others to the temptation to cheat because they are often operating with a handicap and feel helpless to win without cheating. Even when they have the opportunity to compete on a more equal basis with other handicapped children, their competitiveness may be enhanced by their hunger, being starved for a chance to win.

These problems are dealt with in three ways: (1) firmly limiting any cheating while interpreting the hunger behind it (for example, "You must really want to win badly in order even to be willing to cheat to do it"); (2) reducing the emphasis on competition by focusing the activities of the children's group on noncompetitive activities in which everyone can feel successful (however, some competitive activities are included so that the children can learn how to deal with that situation); and (3) educating the children in more adaptive, realistic attitudes through discussion, interpretation, advice, brainwashing, and any other means available. The following example illustrates the application of the third approach just after the children had returned from their separate group:

Dr. A.: OK, who wants to tell us what you did? [Several hands raise.] OK, Ron?

Ron: We played relays and kickball.

Dr. A.: Relays and kickball. Was there anything else?

Ron: Crabball!

Dr. A.: Crabball? What is crabball?

Kurt: I know . . .

Dr. A.: OK, what is it?

Kurt: Well, it's where you sit on your back like this (*demonstrating*) and kick the ball.

Dr. A.: Oh, you get in the shape of a crab. That sounds like it would be hard to do.

Kurt: Yeh, for us boys, but not for Mrs. S. Yeah, they won all the games because they got to pick 'em. I said I wanted to play crawl and she said "no" (*bitingly*) cuz she didn't want to get her pants dirty. [Laughter from the rest of the group.] That's why I said crawling so that way we could win . . .

Dr. A.: Oh, you were going to use unfair tactics?

Kurt: Billie and Mrs. S. were the only ones good at what they picked.

Mrs. S.: Well, Kurt, I don't know if it's quite like that. I think that you guys were pretty good at it and won quite a few relays also. I think it was about even.

Kurt: (*counting out loud*) One, two, three, four, five.

Dr. A.: What was it? Boys against girls?

Kurt: Yeh.

Billie: It was Mrs. S., the medical student, and me against the boys.

Dr. A.: Oh, I see. Are you saying the teams weren't even?

Kurt: The teams weren't fair because they took bigger steps (*referring to Mrs. S. and the medical student*) when they was running.

Medical student: Well, Kurt, we're a lot bigger and older.

Dr. A.:   Yeh, Kurt, they're over the hill. [Laughter.] It sounds like, Kurt, that the only way to make it fair would be for you to win all the games.

Kurt: No, for us to win one or two games.

Mrs. S.
and Billie: You did!

Kurt: I mean about five or six. [Laughter from the rest.]

Mrs. S.:   You mean five or six games out of eight?

Dr. A.:   How many games were there?

Kurt: About eight.

Dr. A.:   You mean you should win about five or six games out of eight?

Kurt: Yep.

Dr. A.:   Well, how many times would that let the other people win?

Ron: Twice. That's how many times they only let us win.

Dr. A.:   Billie, what do you think about this?

Billie: I don't think it's fair.

Kurt: That's because you're a girl.

Billie: Right.

Dr. A.:   Billie, would you think it's fair if you were the one that won five or six games and the others only two?

Billie: No.

Dr. A.:   You wouldn't? What would be fair?

Billie: If both sides were equal.

Dr. A.:   You say both sides should have about equal wins?

Kurt: (*annoyed*) You call that equal to us?

Dr. A.: Well, what would you call equal, Kurt?

Kurt: Well, I guess even.

Dr. A.: You mean four games a piece?

Kurt: Yeah.

Dr. A.: Well, you said that you wanted to win five or six games. You said that would be fair.

Kurt and
Tom: That would be fair. (*grinning*)

Dr. A.: OK, Ron, what do you think would be fair? To have your team win five or six and the other team only two or three or for each side to win four? What would be fair?

Ron: To win all of them.

Dr. A.: Oh, you want to win all of them! And the other side none! You think that would be fair?

Mrs. S.: I don't think you know what fair means.

Dr. A.: Is that what you guys think is fair? For you guys to win 'em all? What do you think Tom?

Tom: (*after a few minutes*) That each team should win the same.

Dr. A.: Oh, you're saying four and four, that each team should win four. That's what Billie said, too. Ron thinks that his team should win eight games and the other side none, that would be fair, and Kurt, are you still saying five or six against two or three, or are you saying four and four? What are you saying?

Kurt: I'm saying at least four.

Dr. A.: You mean four on one team and four on the other?

Kurt: Yep.

Dr. A.: Why do you think Ron said that it would be fair for you to win all the games and the other side none? Why would he say that would be fair?

Kurt: Cuz we haven't won once.

Dr. A.: You mean that would make up for the times that you didn't win any?

Kurt: Right.

Dr. A.: OK, but Ron hasn't been in the group before. So he wouldn't know about the times that you didn't win. Kurt, you said you thought each team should win four, right? That would be fair. Three of you kids said it would be fair for each team to win four games, but Ron said the only thing that would be fair is for his team to win eight and the other team none. Why do you think he would say something like that?

Billie: I don't think he knows what *fair* means. [Note Billie's imitation of Mrs. S.]

Dr. A.: Yes, his idea of fair is for him to win everything and the other side to win nothing. The rest of you said it was fair for each side to win half. What do you think is the difference between the way Ron is thinking and the rest of you are thinking?

Billie: Well, I guess I would like to win all of them, too.

Dr. A.: Yes, that's the way you'd like it to be, to win all of them, but you realize that wouldn't be fair. Right? [Billie nods.] You know that what's fair and what you'd like may be two different things: that it's fair for each side to win half, but what you'd like to do is to win them all. So maybe he's not making a difference between what's fair and what he wants.

Dr. A. is orchestrating a lot of pressure, both peer pressure and implied authority opinion, on Ron. It is important to mention the nonverbal communication that keeps this pressure constructive because such intentional pressure on one youngster in a group could be destructive, including the possibility of scapegoating. Throughout this discussion, Dr. A.'s gestures and tone of voice implied a respect for the opinions of all the children, including Ron. Dr. A. implied that Ron must have a good reason for taking his deviant position and that if the rest of the group could understand his reasons, they would be empathetic. At no point was Ron directly told that he should change his opinion, but the discussion was structured in such a way as to suggest the right answers to him and provide an easy way for him to shift to the correct opinion. This is an application of the "big truth" technique. Note also how the pressure on Ron is titrated by twice diverting the discussion to other people when Ron seems overwhelmed and then bringing the focus back to him again when he seems able to handle it.

Dr. A.:	Maybe to him being fair means to give him what he wants. What about that, Ron; could that be it? Were you kind of making those two things the same? What you want and what's fair: do you think those are the same thing? [There is no response from Ron.] It's not the same thing, is it? Maybe we can get some help from the grown-ups in understanding this because it's kind of an important thing. In fact, this is what the parents were talking about a little bit in their group: how maybe somebody wants something so much that they think it's not fair if they don't get everything? It's not fair if I don't win all the games, or it's not fair if I don't get all the presents; it's not fair if I don't get whatever I want or if somebody else gets something. That can happen, you know. People can get to think that way. Maybe some of the adults can help us by telling us how they worked it out. Because they grew up already, they can tell how they got to learn the difference between what's fair and what I want.
Billie's mother (Mrs. V.):	Well, in any game there is always a winner and a loser. Everyone can't always win, and you can learn good sportsmanship this way.

Dr. A. invited contributions from the adults to set a good example for the children and to clarify with concrete examples the point he had been trying to develop. Such an invitation to the parents also helps the children see their parents as resource people in resolving problems. In this instance, the parent's response was not along the lines anticipated but turned out to be a useful tangent, which Dr. A. opportunistically explored:

Dr. A.:	So you mean even when you lose, you can get something out of it because you can learn to be a good sport?
Children:	Yes.

Dr. A.:   You can make friends even when you're losing. That's a good thought. Does anybody here want to make more friends?

Kurt: Yes!

Dr. A.:   Would you like to have more friends Ron? Billie? Tom? [All nod except Ron.]

Ron: I already have too many.

Dr. A.:   Oh, you have too many friends! That explains it! I guess a good way to get rid of some of them is to beat them all the time. Is that really what you want to do—get rid of friends? [Ron looks bewildered.] Does anyone else have any ideas about the difference between what you want and what's fair? Are there any other advantages to being a good sport? To not winning all the games . . . to winning at least half of the games?

Ron: Well, in school this one class in basketball beats us all the time. The score was 7 to 0.

Dr. A.:   Do you think its fair that they beat you all the time? [Ron shakes his head.] What would you think if they said it's fair for us to beat you all the time—to win all the games? What do you think about that?

Ron: I would tell Mr. Rutter, the gym teacher.

Ron is ten years old but still seems to be exhibiting egocentric thinking: the inability to see things from another person's viewpoint. This is part of a general immaturity, but because he is of normal intelligence, there is reasonable hope that at this age he can be nudged into a more concrete-operational type of thinking rather than egocentric. If he were below age six, it would not be advisable to attempt to get him to see the other person's viewpoint. At the younger age, fairness would have to be dealt with on a "one for you, one for me, one for you" basis).

Dr. A.:   What do you think about this idea: they are winning all the games, and your class is not winning any of them. They want to beat you all the time. What would you say if they said, "It's fair for us to win all the games"?

Ron: I would say that's not fair.

Dr. A.: Well, what's the difference between them saying "it's fair for us to win all the games," and you saying, "it's fair for us to win all the games"? Is it fair for you to win all the games if it's not fair for them to win all the games?

Ron: No.

Dr. A.: That's good. You have learned something about what we have talked about.

Billie: It would be fair if they practice before all the games.

Dr. A.: Oh, you're saying it would be fair for somebody to win all the games because they deserved to win, because they work harder. [Ron shakes his head.] Ron's not agreeing. He says that even if one team practices and works harder, it's still not fair for them to win all the games. Is that what you are saying?

Ron: They still win and they don't even practice. They cheat.

Here Ron demonstrates again his difficulty of operating on the same conceptual level as Billie, his age peer. Despite his brief breakthrough into operational thinking, he reverts again to egocentric thinking and interprets Billie's comment as referring to his situation rather than things in general. If time permitted, it might pay to explore this problem, but with time running out, Dr. A. chose to redirect the focus to Billie's point:

Dr. A.: But do you think the team that practices harder should win more?

Ron: Yes.

When the point is stated clearly and simply, Ron is able to see it and agree to it. He adapted much more quickly in the second instance to the suggestions of the other child. In succeeding sessions, Ron conformed more and more to the standards of the group and became more realistic in his expectations. The group in general, especially Kurt, developed more helpfulness and cooperation in place of competition and cries of unfairness.

13
Sibling Relations

E ver since Cain and Abel, siblings have vied for parental favors and compared themselves invidiously. One of the underlying myths perpetuating sibling strife is the belief that whatever one sibling has—material goods, parental love, personal abilities—is at the expense of another. Sibling rivalry is not a necessary state of affairs but is often inadvertently precipitated by misguided parental efforts to treat all their children equally and to feel guilty if they do not satisfy all of their children's desires.

Learning- and behavior-disordered children and their siblings are particularly vulnerable to feelings of sibling competition because of the handicapped child's immaturity, insecurity, low self-esteem, poor impulse control, troublesomeness to other members of the family, and consumption of disproportionate parental attention and resources. In addition, behavior-disordered children are especially vulnerable to scapegoating. Sibling relation problems are thus manifested in two major ways: the bottomless pit competition for parental attention and the attempt to shore up self-esteem and find a secure family role by assigning and accepting "good guy" and "bad guy" roles.

This chapter presents excerpts from two groups, one from a parents' segment and one embracing both a parents' segment and combined parent and child segment.

Oral Rivalry

Here is an excerpt of parents discussing their children's apparent jealousy of one another. Some of the parents experience great relief and comfort from learning that another parent's child had similar problems to their own child's. Mrs. T. had just reported valiant but unsuccessful efforts to deal with the problem of insatiable, excessive demands.

Dr. A.:   It sounds like you've done a lot of things right. As you talk, I recall some of the things Mrs. E. mentioned last week. It seems like you deserve to have better results than you do. I don't think you should give up on what you're doing because it didn't seem to work or because one child didn't respond the way you expected. All you can do is decide what you can give and that's it. They'll always want more. Give what you can freely once you decide what you want to give, so there isn't any cajoling or coaxing for more or so they don't feel you are begrudging them. Maybe, Mrs. E., you can share some things about Kurt.

Mrs. E.: Well, if you spent the whole day with Kurt alone and he found out Tom or Sally got a candy bar, then that was it. That was more than anything you did the whole day with Kurt. Even though you took him to the zoo, it didn't matter.

Mr. V.: I can understand what you are saying, Mrs. E. Billie is very jealous too, for no reason. You see, Billie was jealous of her sister Ilene's diet. She had a very serious enzyme problem resulting in a special diet. The first couple of years of her diet, she could eat only rice, soybeans, Jello, and soy milk. She was not allowed to eat any milk products. What we decided on was that Billie could have the same diet as Ilene if she wanted. But that didn't stop the jealousy.

Mrs. E.: Yes, I know how it is. You can try so hard, and it won't make a difference. Around Christmas time, we offered to get Kurt a new coat if he would give Tom his old one, but he refused. I couldn't understand it. You would think a child would rather have something new, but that wasn't the case.

Dr. E.: What age was Billie when you tried this diet?

Mr. V.: She was about two and a half.

Dr. E.: She might understand now even though she didn't then. A child under age six cannot understand another person's viewpoint. Even a very bright child cannot understand another person's point of view before age six. They will always act as if everyone knows what they know. They will tell you a story leaving out important points and expect you to know what they are talking about.

Dr. A.: That's right. They can't seem to appreciate the other side. If you ask them to tell you what the other side of the room looks like, they can't until they walk over to that side of the room. They can't move things around in their mind. They can't appreciate your side. All Billie knows, for example, is that Ilene got Jello and she didn't. All Kurt knows is that Tom or Sally got ice cream and he didn't. It is irrelevant to Billie that she got to eat things that the other didn't. I bet that she understands it now. She may choose not to understand, or she doesn't want to. That's an emotional problem. There may be some advantage in doing that. At this point she should be capable of it though. At least you know she has the ability. I don't know when Kurt began to see the viewpoint of others. He has become more accepting, though.

Mrs. E.: He didn't completely stop. He still has some problems with it. I can't really place a time on it. It was real bad when Kurt was in kindergarten, and I was just home with Tom. If Kurt found out that we got an ice cream cone, that would be it for the rest of the week. In the last six months to a year, he's done better.

Dr. A.: Has Ron shown jealousy of his sister?

Mrs. Q.: Every once in a while. He shows more jealousy of his real sister than two stepsisters. Amazing, isn't it? He wants to be allowed to do the same things as them.

Mr. V.: We get that, too.

Dr. A.: Maybe he considers his stepsiblings more like friends and doesn't feel as threatened by them because they don't have the same claim on you as full sibs. If he could feel more secure, he might treat his sister as well as his stepsisters.

Mrs. Q.: Maybe we can get him to be friends with his sister.

The Good Guys and the Bad Guys

The following week, the same topic persisted, in a modified form. We pick it up in the middle of parents' group:

Mrs. E.: Things have been really going bad this week. Kurt and Tom are fighting something terrible. I just don't know what to do. This morning they were fighting so bad that I said something I shouldn't have said because I didn't stick to it. I threatened that they would miss therapy today. But I didn't know whether to bring them or let them stay home because it's so important to come here.

Dr. A.:   It sounds like you're feeling bad because you didn't live up to the demands you had set. You feel bad you didn't carry out the threat, but also you feel bad because you would have deprived them of therapy. It sounds like you didn't feel confident with the system. [The previous week, Mrs. E. had decided if Kurt and Tom misbehaved getting ready, they would have to miss group.]

Mrs. D.:   It worked for Mannie.

Dr. A.:   It may be different for Mannie. With Mannie, he would come here for a while and do fine. Then his parents said he didn't have to come. He would misbehave in order to come here, so I reversed the situation. When he was good, he got to come; when he was bad, he didn't get to come. Maybe, Mrs. E., you can try alternating weeks. Bring one child on one week, the other on the opposite week. If they both behave, they can both come. In this way they'll learn if they cooperate, they can both come.

Dr. E.:   (*to Mrs. V., Paul's mother, a new member of the parents' group*) How is it with one boy and all sisters at home? How do they get along?

Mrs. V.:   He [Paul] used to get all the attention.

Dr. E.:   That could be misleading. He may come to think that the rest of the world is going to treat him just as special.

Mrs. E.:   Kurt has the opposite problem. Instead of Sally giving him special attention, he tries to get his older sister's goat. This week he showed his butt to Sally, and now she's beginning to resent him. She used to favor him. But now since he is so bad and gets all this special treatment, she really resents him.

Dr. E.:   What do you mean?

Mrs. E.:   Well, Kurt brags a lot to her about coming here and all the things he does in school. It's a private boys' school, you know, so they have a lot of extracurricular activities set up for the boys. She doesn't understand why he gets to do all this stuff when he's so bad.

Dr. E.:   It sounds like a legitimate complaint on her part. Have you ever thought about setting up some time to do special things with Sally so she feels that her good behavior is noticed or that it's worth continuing?

Mrs. E.: Well, I thought I was doing that. But Kurt and Tom try to ruin it all the time. They act up right before we leave, and by the time we leave I'm in such a rotten mood that I can hardly enjoy Sally.

Dr. E.: I think it's important that Sally gets her special time. No matter how difficult it is, you should ignore the boys at this time. It sounds like a manipulation on their part.

Dr. A.: I'm curious about this mooning. It is a thing with teenagers, but I'm not sure what the payoff is for Kurt.

Mrs. E.: Well, she screams and yells. By making a fuss, she probably reinforces him. [Mrs. E. is demonstrating some behavior management principles she has learned from attending the group. Note how she only needs the question posed to apply the principle she has learned.]

Dr. A.: Has anyone else had this problem?

Mrs. T.: Not the mooning problem, but Penny is constantly aggravating her older sister, whom I don't have a problem with.

Dr. A.: It sounds like in each family situation described so far there is a good guy and a bad guy.

Mrs. T.: That sounds like you have something there. It's true. When Irene gets reprimanded, Penny becomes good.

Dr. A.: Is it possible that Irene is good all the time because you're always on Penny?

Mrs. T.: I'm not sure. I feel we treat them the same, and they both behave so differently, so it's kind of hard to tell.

Dr. E.: Is it possible that Irene gets something out of the negative attention you're always giving to Penny?

Mrs. T.: Well, I never really ever thought of it that way.

At this moment the children returned from their group. Think how you would adapt the parents' conversation to the children's participation. With which point would you lead into the children's discussion? Here is the way it actually was handled.

Dr. A.: You kids would be interested to hear what the parents talked about. We talked about how in some families there is a good guy and a bad guy. Does anybody here know what I mean when I say good guy and bad guy? [Laughter from the children.] Why do you think that happens?

Kurt: We fight a lot in our family.

Dr. A.: Oh. Who else fights a lot in their family? [Each child affirmed fights with their families.] What makes a kid a bad guy? Can anyone tell me what a bad guy does?

Paul: Being a bully.

Dr. A.: Oh, that's right. If you're a bully, then maybe someone would think you're a bad guy. In your family, Paul, are you a good guy or bad guy?

Paul: I do what my mom tells me to do.

Dr. A.: How do you tell the difference between a good guy and a bad guy?

Paul: You listen.

Dr. A.: How do you know you've listened?

Kurt: If he gets swats, he's a bad guy.

Dr. A.: How do you know how many swats make a good or bad guy?

Kurt: Three swats, you're a good guy; four swats, you're a bad guy.

Dr. A.: All right, how many of you have a good guy or a bad guy in your family? [Each child nodded he or she had one.]

Tom: Kurt's the bad guy in our family.

Dr. A.: Well, Tom, what are you if Kurt's the bad guy? I see that you're smiling. [No response.] Does anyone here compare themselves to someone else? Does anyone here think they're a good guy if they do better than everyone else? Can everyone be a good guy? Kurt? Tom? Penny? Paul? [No response from the children.] How could you know if you were a good guy if there is no bad guy in the family? Is it possible for everyone to be a good guy?

Penny: If you mind your mother . . .

Dr. A.: Suppose you minded 95 percent of the time, and your sister minds 100 percent of the time. Would you be a bad guy?

Penny: No, she would be the bad guy . . .

Dr. A.: The thing that I am wondering about is that if it makes a kid better when there is somebody worse.

Paul: I like to be worse so my cousins teach me new things. They pick me up and pass me around.

Think how you would handle this off-the-wall response. Actually we handled it by ignoring it, but would like to suggest the following two better alternatives: question the implied causal connection—"How does being worse get your cousins to teach you new things?"—or interpret the implied assumption: "It's sounds like you think you have to be a bad guy to keep your cousins interested in you" or "Would your cousins still like you if you were a good guy?"

Dr. A.: What I'd like you kids to figure out this week for a homework assignment is a way to tell whether you're a good guy or a bad guy without comparing yourself to other kids. Maybe you can talk to your mother about how you can be a good guy without comparing yourself to the other kids. I think it is possible for everyone to be a good guy, but it's too hard when you compare yourself to another kid.

Dr. E.: I think its important for the kids to know that there will always be somebody somewhere who is better and worse than you by a little. But that's not so important. What is most important is if you can be a little better than you were last week. That's what makes a good guy.

14
Peer Relations, Self-Determination, and Reputation

Even adults are concerned about what family, friends, and colleagues think of them. We all want to be liked or at least accepted. This often poses a conflict: we must choose between pleasing someone else and respecting our own needs, beliefs, and principles. Throughout life we are repeatedly confronted with such decisions. To what degree will our concern for our reputation and our desire to be liked and respected influence how we behave? Will we sell out to be liked, or will we adhere to behavior of our own choice?

Young children may not have yet developed the mental structures to make such a decision logically. They think intuitively and concretely and sometimes behave impulsively. Children with learning or behavior problems or other handicaps have particular difficulty. They already lack confidence, security, and feelings of acceptance. Both their academic inadequacy and social clumsiness contribute to feelings of inadequacy. They often have difficulty keeping friends. This makes them especially sensitive to the issues of reputation and role. Sometimes, to maintain a semblance of acceptance, a child may yield to peer pressure to sustain a clown, scapegoat, troublemaker, or other negative role or reputation.

Living Down a Bad Reputation

In a parents' group, Mrs. B., Robert's mother, brought up her concern about Robert's bad reputation from the previous school year. She explained that during second grade, he began to receive failing grades and was becoming a behavior problem at home and school. He was sent to the office often and sent home several times. During the first week of the new school year (third grade), he was called into the principal's office and told he had one more chance, even though this year he had not yet been in any trouble. Mrs. B. expressed her concern that Robert was being labeled a problem and was not being given a fair, fresh start. According to Mrs. B., it was apparent that the principal was basing this warning on the past. She felt intimidated by the principal, although she did not speak to him about Robert. He had made her feel as if Robert was the only troublesome child. Several parents urged Mrs. B. to communicate with Robert's teacher and principal.

After the children returned from their separate group, the parents' topic was adapted to the children's discussion:

Dr. A.: Did anyone in here ever hear of the word *reputation*?

Dan: Yeah; it's what other people think of you—good, smart, or dumb.

Craig: It's like a career, putting your reputation on the line. They're important, like jobs.

Dr. A.: That's right! Why are reputations important? [Puzzled looks.] How is a reputation important in terms of friends? [Blank stares.] Why is a bad reputation not good? Could it mean that you'll get a whipping for something you didn't do? [Kurt nods.] Does that ever happen to any of you? [All the children raise their hands.] It's hard to work out of a bad reputation, isn't it? How can you get out of a bad reputation?

Sarah: You can just be good.

Dr. A.: When you start, do you think people will believe you? [The children look indecisive.] You may have a hard time convincing people! What if someone says they are going to reform and they don't?

Craig: You get in worse trouble because then people will never believe you.

Dr. E.: That's right! How long do you think it will take before people will believe you?

Kurt: About two days.

Tom: About a week.

Sarah: A half a year if you're in deep trouble.

Dr. E.: That's right; it may take some time to convince other people.

Dr. A.: What do you have to take from other people until you prove it? [The children look bewildered.] Well, I think you should know that there will probably be some people who will try to keep you with a bad reputation—like other kids in school. They have to have someone to blame.

Dr. E.: Other people may try to do things to trick you into a bad reputation. It will take time to convince people, and you have to continue to be good for a long time to get rid of it.

Kurt: (*smirking*) Maybe you don't want to get rid of it.

On reviewing the transcript of this session, Dr. A. was surprised to note this last comment by Kurt. He did not hear it in the live session and was chagrined at having missed an opportunity that he would have liked to have used like this:

Dr. A.: That's an important point, Kurt. Do the rest of you understand what he said? I think I do. I think he's talking about how hard it is to change from a bad guy to a good guy inside and how sometimes the idea of changing is so scary that maybe a kid thinks it's better to keep on being a bad guy rather than take a chance. It seems safer to keep on having a bad reputation; at least then you're somebody, and you know who you are. Besides, maybe the people who know you would rather you stay the same. They may get upset if you don't live up to your bad reputation. It kind of comes down to whether you're going to be man enough to take a chance and become a good guy or whether you're going to give in to the pressure of what other people expect you to do. So I'm glad you brought that up, Kurt. What do you other kids think about it?

Making and Keeping Friends

Toward the end of a parents' group, Mrs. Q. expressed a concern that her son repeatedly says he is the dumbest child in the class and nobody likes him. Mrs. Q. claimed that he had always done well in school, and his academic failure now is probably a result of his social maladjustment.

Dr. A.: Mrs. Q., are you in the situation where you see him making progress, but it seems like the problem is getting worse because his age-mates are growing further ahead?

Mrs. Q.: That may be. When he comes home from school after a bad day, he's in such a bad mood. He's angry, but he doesn't express it. He does say, "Nobody likes me." He leaves work in school to talk to others; then he never finishes his work. I just think if he solved his social problems, his academics would improve. I think his visits are an attempt to make friends.

Dr. A.: Sounds like he is defeating his own purpose by turning off the other kids. Has anyone talked with him about defeating his own purpose?

Mrs. Q.: Yes, and he denies that he even does it.

Dr. A.: Perhaps he needs a specific plan for what he can do. When a child decides on something he wants to change, he should have a plan so he won't do the same thing again.

This direct advice by Dr. A. was a bit rushed and premature, but the children could be heard in the distance returning to the room and there was not time for a more appropriate cultivation of the issue. After the children returned and described their groups, the discussion continued:

Dr. A.: Has anyone ever heard the words *second fiddle friend*? [The children look interested and expectant.] Does it ever happen to anyone where you want someone to be your best friend, but he'll only play with you when his other friends are not around?

Tom: That happened to me.

Dr. A.: Has that ever happened to you, Kurt?

Kurt: No.

Dr. A.: Have you ever done that to someone else?

Kurt: No.

Dr. A.: Sometimes the people doing it don't realize it. Is it possible for all three to be friends? [The children shrug.] Why is it important to have friends?

Rich Y.: You'd be lonely.

Dr. A.: What about your brothers and sisters? [The children frown on mention of sisters.] They're not your friends?

Rich P.:   My sister is weird.

Dr. A.:   Can anyone else tell me why it is important to have friends? [The children appear anxious.] It's something you can do all your life. Adults have friends. Let's find out from your mothers why they think it's important to have friends.

Kurt: (*interrupting sarcastically*) So they can get you out of the house and so they have time to themselves. [Laughter from the adults.]

There are several options in response to Kurt's half-humorous cynical comment: (1) use it as an opportunity to discuss the need for adults (and children) to have some privacy; (2) use it as an opportunity to discuss mutual respect; (3) use it as an opportunity to discuss feelings of neglect or rejection; (4) use it as an opportunity to discuss rights and duties of parents and children and perhaps human limitations of parents (Kurt is always critical of his parents); (5) ignore the comment to avoid reinforcing such verbal behavior and continue with the original topic or set limits by restating that it is the parents' turn to answer. Any of these is acceptable. Dr. A. actually chose number 5, but this does not imply that it is any better than the others.

Dr. A.:   Let's ask the mothers.

Mrs. P.:   I think it's important to have friends because you learn to trust and you learn how to get along with other people.

Several other parents continued a discussion of the importance of friends and how to make and keep them, providing an opportunity for the children to see their parents as a resource.

15

Responsibility: Who Owns It?

Responsibility, like its counterpart, accountability, is an awesome concept. It is both attractive and frightening. It has implications of maturity and autonomy but also of vulnerability to blame, drudgery, and boredom. Parents (and often teachers) often describe a child as lacking responsibility. Such parents often are unwittingly reinforcing the child's failure to become responsible by taking responsibility for him or her. Children may see themselves as unprivileged and oversupervised but fail to see that the pathway to privilege and freedom is through demonstrating responsibility. They are quite happy to allow their parents to continue responsibility for things that they themselves could begin assuming responsibility for.

Parents are not in a favorable position to enlighten the child in this regard, partly because they do not always see the picture clearly themselves and partly because the issues of responsibility are usually colored by such intense previous parent-child struggles, frustrations, disappointments, and resentment that it is hard for either parent or child to be rational about it. Furthermore, children are likely to interpret their parents' attempts to explain the allures of responsibility as an attempt to seduce them into doing work or making life easier for the parent. As in so many other things, children will often accept from a more neutral person ideas that they would reject from their parents. Consequently responsibility is an important topic for discussion with both parents and children. This chapter shows examples of such discussion from four different sessions: one example from a combined children's and parents' segment of a group, two from the separate parents' segment, and one example overlapping between a separate parents' segment and the combined segment.

Explaining and Selling Responsibility

After the children returned from their separate group, the topic was adapted to their participation:

Dr. A.:   The parents have been talking about something very important: responsibility. One of the things that came up was homework. [Groans from the children.] They have the impression that you kids don't like homework. Is that right? [Laughter from the whole group while Dr. A., with tongue in cheek, asks each of the children in turn, and each affirms a dislike of homework. Humor assists in programming the children to respond affirmatively. Starting the discussion with some questions, either serious or joking, that invite an obvious "yes" answer helps the youngsters develop a habit of agreeing and confidence in responding. This programming is helpful preparation for their acceptance and affirmation of less obvious ideas later in the session.] Whose responsibility is it for you to pass in school: is it the mother's, father's or the kids'? Tom, what do you think?

Tom: I think it's the mother's.

Mannie: Both parents' and kids'.

Kurt: Parents'.

Sandra: Mother.

Think about how you could respond. The children are not following a desired script; they say it's the parents' responsibility. How would you circumvent the danger of overtly disagreeing with the child? One way is to accept the children's statements as how things are at home rather than how they ought to be. One can then question again with the implication that although the children's original opinions were accepted, a different answer is called for to describe how things should be.

Dr. A.:   Who do you think should be responsible? Who should be more interested in the homework? [Each of the children in turn, when asked, asserted that the parents should be more interested. The children have still not read the script. The therapist by this time is feeling some urgency to convince them that they should be more interested than the parents. Instead he reverses roles and invites the children to convince him.] Can you kids convince me that the parents should be more interested in homework? Why should they?

Kurt: Because if you get good grades, you can get a good job and make money for your parents. [Laughter from group.]

Mannie: [Mannie had been in a passive-aggressive feud with his parents over schoolwork.] Well, I guess the kids should be more concerned because your parents can't get your grades up. You end up hurting yourself to hurt your parents.

Dr. A.:   How many kids or adults have hurt yourself to hurt someone else? Like not doing something for your own good just because somebody else wants you to do it? [All nod their heads.] I guess the point is for you kids to feel good about doing things that are for your own good.

Kurt: [Kurt had been chronically depressed in a hostile, sour, punishing manner.] Is this like not wanting to feel good so your mother won't feel good?

Dr. A.:   Yes, Kurt, that's it.

The message to the children regarding responsibility was detoxified by having it addressed as part of a peer group, having the therapist discuss it rather than the parents, carefully avoiding putting down the children's responses, and using the technique of restating the question with further challenge, which suggests to the children that their response was not complete. The children seemed quick to grasp that responsibility is for one's own benefit more than for the parents'. Note the amount of constructive insight these children were able to volunteer when respectfully and cordially challenged to examine their reasons for their opinion. Perhaps this observation was not lost on the parents.

Teaching Parents How to Pass the Buck

Here is an excerpt of a parents' discussion on the topic of responsibility:

Dr. A.:   *(to Tom's father, Mr. E.)* Last time you were here, we had talked about Kurt and Tom carrying out their assignments and your dissatisfaction with what they had chosen. How do you feel about their assignments now?

Mr. E.:   With Tom cleaning his room, he had to be reminded by Kurt and myself. Some days Tom just spaces out and doesn't do his work, and some days he does it.

Dr. E.:   Do you have any ideas as to why this is so? [Although the leaders had ideas about how Tom was carrying out his assignment, they first invited the parent to express his opinion and then gradually build the interpretation.]

Mr. E.:   No, I'm really not sure.

Dr. A.:   Is he maybe doing a better job than he lets on? Often Tom appears to not have done any of his assignment, and then Kurt reports that he had actually cleaned part of his room.

Dr. E.:   Yes, that is a change of behavior for Kurt. He usually says something negative about Tom, and this time he helped Tom out of a fix.

Mr. E.:   Wasn't he supposed to bring a chart in last week?

Dr. A.:   Yes, I think so, but he didn't bring it in.

Mr. E.:   Yes, there is a chart on his door, and he said he made it in school.

Dr. E.:   As you recall, his goal was to clean part of his room at a time.

Mr. E.:   Well, I had to get on him or else he wouldn't do it.

Dr. A.:   But Kurt claimed that he had cleaned some of it.

Mr. E.:   I don't know why he acts like he doesn't know what's going on, like a baby.

Dr. A.:   Maybe a good assignment will be to say something good about himself.

Dr. E.:   Seems that both Kurt and Tom have molded their roles. At home they fit into the expectations people have of them. Then when they come here, they have another set of expectations placed on them. I was kind of wondering what Tom's responsibility was in all of this. Is it possible not to remind Tom to do things he has to do? (*referring to Mr. E.*) What bothers me is that he has chosen an assignment, and he has managed to get you and Kurt to do it for him, as well as report it for him. He needs to take the initiative.

Dr. A.:   Yes, that's a line of thinking that some adults have problems with as well. If they can blame someone else, then it's not their fault.

They get someone else to take the responsibility. For example, in Tom's case, he simply forgets to ask the teacher for the paper, or he says he doesn't see any paper in school. What happens next is that you and Kurt supply what he didn't do for himself. You supply the reminder. He then comes in here and doesn't report what he did—that he did part of the job himself. He even gets Kurt to report it for him. So he's always getting someone else to speak for him and do things for him. It's kind of like a passive recipient. It's very hard to deal with because the natural tendency is to push or move him along. Of course, sometimes you may have to do that if you have to go somewhere and be somewhere at a certain time.

Dr. E.: Sometimes there is no choice, but sometimes there is a choice.

Dr. A.: The problem is your natural urge in wanting to push. If he is going to be an immovable object, you're going to be an irresistable force. The problem is that it is so efficient, easy, and effective to just do nothing. The Rock of Gibraltar has stood for centuries, and all the irresistible forces—the waves, the storms, the winds— have beat on it and haven't accomplished anything because all it has to do is just sit there. It's a very efficient role to just sit there like a Rock of Gibraltar. It doesn't take any energy. You are at a disadvantage if you try to fight him on his own terms, that is, if you get into pushing him to do something he won't do for himself. I think it's kind of hopeless. I advise you to give it up. That's hard to do.

Dr. E.: Giving up or not pushing him is something different than you've done before since he is so used to having everyone do everything for him. He needs to learn to take the consequences himself for his own behavior. We would have to deal with it in here.

Mrs. K.: [She has been in a passive-aggressive feud with Billie with her math assignments.] How can you not push them on things they're supposed to do, that any normal kid should do? It's very difficult for the parents to just sit there and take it.

Dr. A.: Yes, it's very difficult to do because the natural inclination is to push, and it does take a long time for them to get hooked on being more active. You can't expect a problem that has taken years to develop to disappear overnight. Only with patience and consistency will the change eventually occur.

Mr. E.: The interesting thing about Tom is that he works around the house with his mother.

Dr. E.: Oh, you mean he enjoys working with someone else?

Mr. E.: Yes, he'll work around the house for hours as long as someone else is right there with him.

Dr. A.: One technique is to at first ask if they would like your help in completing a task. Help them with the chore, and then the next time let them know it is their responsibility, but you will help if they need it. In this manner, you are gradually fading yourself out and giving them more of the responsibility. Oftentimes kids are afraid of doing something for the first time. They may lack the confidence.

Reinforcing the Lesson

A few months later in the parents' group, Mr. E. brought up his dissatisfaction with Kurt's performance in school. While waiting for an appointment with Kurt's teacher, Mr. E. constructively consulted with Kurt on the matter. Note how Mr. E. used what he had learned from previous sessions.

Mr. E.: I plainly said to Kurt, "This was a slip from what you started off. I don't understand why this has happened. Why do you think this has happened?" Well, Kurt didn't respond, but the next week for his group assignment, he picked improving his grades.

Dr. A.: I guess one of the encouraging things is that Kurt picked an assignment that wasn't just trivial. It shows that he does care about it and wants to do something worthwhile. This is a good example of how a child often ends up doing exactly what you want him to do if you don't pressure or push him.

Mr. E.: He said he was going to make an effort. We didn't have to say a whole lot about it.

Dr. A.: It seems like you handled that well with the attitude you took. You made a little suggestion or encouragement, no anger or coercion, just kind of consulting with him. [Note that Dr. A. is reinforcing the parent. Also, by repeating the desirable methods the parent used, he raised the consciousness of the desirable concepts for all the parents present. Watch what happens.]

Mr. E.: I wanted to make clear that it was his responsibility and that it was something he should be working on and that this is something that

I wasn't going to police. I guess if you can draw them into the idea of cooperation and taking responsibility, that's the best way to go. [This is exactly what the therapist had said the previous month. Often it takes the parents time, just as it does the child, to assimilate and use the concepts.] My wife and I could be screaming and yelling, "This is what you are gonna do, and you're not going to do this for the next six weeks." This is what I got when I was a child, and it certainly didn't make me want to do better. Certainly if I did better, it was only because I was so angry that was the only way to let it out. I don't know; I just handle them the way I would want to be handled, especially if I were a child. When I was a child, I didn't feel like I ever had a choice.

Dr. E.: Do you feel sometimes because of the strictness that you were brought up with and resented that it is hard for you to lay down the law at home?

Mr. E.: When it gets to that point where I have the choice of really being hard, I would much rather reason with them to get their cooperation.

Dr. A.: I think it's a pretty fortunate age that you started working on these things. They are old enough to begin to take responsibility yet young enough to still teach them.

Mr. E.: I can remember back when I was a boy, I think some of the problems I had were because there was no communication, just orders that were issued.

Dr. E.: Are you saying that how you communicate with the child has an effect on how motivated they will be in taking responsibility?

Mr. E.: Yes, that's it. I wished my feelings had been taken into account when decisions were made. Things would have been a lot different for me.

Dr. A.: I guess there's a difference between taking the kids' feelings into account and letting them make the final decision. It's very important that the children still know who is boss, as well as for the boss to consider their feelings. [This statement was added for the sake of the less assertive parents who have difficulty setting limits.]

During another session one month later, Mrs. E. shared with the other parents her progress in dealing with Kurt's acceptance of responsibility:

Mrs. E.:   I remember how bad it was. We've been coming here for about six months or so [the E's were one of the longer-term group families], and we've kind of worked things out. Just about everything is taken care of at this point.

Dr. E.:   What do you mean you worked it out?

Mrs. E.:   Well, Kurt wouldn't get up in the morning. I used to get him up in the morning, and he wouldn't get up. I would end up some mornings getting him out of bed physically, putting his clothes on, taking his hands and walking him downstairs, and literally shoving his breakfast down his throat. He would be putting all this responsibility on me. By the time I could get up in the morning, I would be a nervous wreck for the rest of the day. Through all of this, he would just yell and screm and fight with me. So what we did for a while was, my husband would go in and tell Kurt it's time to get up. If he didn't get up at once or by the time the bus would come, I would ignore all of his screaming, put his clothes on, take him downstairs, put his coat on, put his lunch box in his hand, and shove him out the door. It took me a long time to ignore the screaming and yelling and not get into it with him. When he'd stay in bed longer than he was supposed to, he wouldn't get any breakfast, of course. He would be taken out of bed, and get right into the cold in the winter. I think, too, when he saw that I wasn't gonna fight with him anymore, somehow he just started taking more of the responsibility himself.

Dr. E.:   The most important thing you did was to hold back from falling into the trap. You did something you never did before.

Mrs. E.:   I would also say when he poked at breakfast, "Well, that's fine, but if you miss the bus, you're walking. Before, I would take him. It took me a long time to realize we don't have to argue about the things they should be doing themselves. Then we will have time to spend to do good things together. Things run pretty smooth now. If the kids start off the day right and everybody does what they're supposed to do, then later on at the end of the day we can do something special. We try to do something special at least once a week. Things run pretty smoothly now. The kids all fix their own breakfast now.

In the middle of this discussion, the children come back from their group and reported on their activities. Then the parents' topic was reintroduced.

Dr. A.: Today we talked about something that maybe you kids never thought about, but it was something that I think you kids ought to know. One of the things that your mothers shared with us is the fact that they worry about you. They worry about you getting things done that you are supposed to do. Does anyone have any ideas about why your mothers worry about you kids? [No response.] Maybe the mothers could share with us some of their thoughts and feelings.

Mrs. P.: Well, I want him [Neal] to understand the difference between right and wrong.

Dr. A.: How does it make you feel when he does something right for himself?

Mrs. P.: It makes me feel good.

Dr. A.: Neal, did you know that? Did you kids know that it makes a mother feel good to see a kid do things for themselves? [Blank stares from the children.] Why do you think a mother would feel good to see a kid do something for himself?

Kurt: (*sarcastically*) So she can do less around the house.

Dr. A.: Is that what you think Kurt? You think your mother is lazy?

Kurt: (*with remorse, realizing how absurd his cutting remark was*) Well, I guess not.

Dr. A.: Maybe some of the other kids have some ideas. Tom? Neal? Billie? What do you think?

Billie: Well, maybe if you do more by yourself, your mom will let you go to the movies or something like that. I don't know.

Dr. A.: Oh, you mean the more you act like a grown-up, the more grown-up things you're allowed to do by yourself?

Billie: Yeah, that's what I mean.

Dr. A.: That's a pretty good idea. I think that's what growing up is all about.

16
Feedback: Does Anyone Really Want It?

Two millenia ago a Greek philosopher counseled, "Know thyself." Since then the human race has been struggling to accomplish that. From humanity's attempt to understand itself eventually emerged the era of self-discovery, honesty, open communication of feelings, feedback, rap sessions, transactional analysis, and weekend encounter groups. But how many normal adults could handle communication and feedback even though they claimed they wanted it? It is small wonder that children have trouble with it.

Although learning- and behavior-disordered children do not usually ask for feedback, it is vital that they receive it and accept it. They suffer inattentiveness and processing problems, with resulting developmental and learning delays in various parameters, including social skills. Impaired in the ability to read nonverbal feedback, these children often misinterpret situations and their transactions with others. They need to learn how to notice and appreciate feedback. Therefore we provide it in the form of words, nonverbal cues, and tangible means (such as the star chart) and repeatedly teach the child the meaning of feedback, its importance, and the necessity of paying attention to it. With this work, we have seen gradual improvement and internalization of feedback.

In the following example, some of the children were already familiar with the idea of feedback from previous groups and could be reinforced for the right answers:

Dr. A.: Today, I'd like to talk with you kids about something very important—something that will be important for the rest of your lives. If you can learn how to pay attention to it and how to take it now when you're still young, you'll have a great advantage. It's something that Mrs. S. gives you every week. Can anyone tell me what it is?

Kurt: [The veteran of the group.] Feedback! (*boldly*)

Dr. A.: Right! Can you tell us what feedback is?

Kurt: It tells you how you're doing.

Dr. A.: That's right, Kurt. (*to the rest of the group*) Feedback is a clue or a tip-off about how you're doing. It could be words like, "That's a good job," or "No, that's wrong," or "You ought to do it this way." It could be another type of feedback, the nonverbal kind, like a smile, a glare, or a special look from somebody. Another kind of feedback is the kind that Mrs. S. gives you, the star charts. They tell you how you're doing in the group. Tell me: what's important about feedback? Why should anybody pay attention to it?

Billie: Because you'll know how good and bad you're doing if you pay attention to it.

Dr. A.: I'm glad you mentioned both kinds of feedback. Good feedback is when somebody tells you the things you did right, like when you get a star or a check on the star chart; bad feedback tells you the things you did wrong, things you shouldn't do. With both kinds of feedback, you know what things to keep on doing and what things to stop doing. Why is that important?

Billie: So you can do better!

Dr. A.: Right! Otherwise, if you want to do better and you don't know what you're supposed to do, how can you do it?

Dr. E.: Does anyone here ever have trouble with feedback, like having a hard time taking it? [Some of the children raise their hands.] What kind of feedback do you have the most trouble with?

Billie: I like to tell other people what they did wrong.

Dr. E.: But do you like it when somebody tells you what you did wrong?

Billie: Yes.

Dr. E.: That's good and quite unusual. Most people have trouble taking it when someone tells them what they did wrong. Then there are others who would rather have someone tell them what they did wrong rather than what they did right. Does anybody here have trouble when somebody tells you something good? Do you ever get embarrassed about it? [Ron smiles.]

Dr. A.: How about you, Ron? Have you ever felt funny when someone tells you something good?

Ron: When I was swimming once and my teacher told me in front of the class that I wasn't doing it right.

Dr. A.: Oh, you mean she told you something negative—something bad? [Ron nods.] That is what is called negative feedback. Are you saying it's kind of hard to take when other people are around? [Ron nods.] You know a little trick for that? When somebody's telling your mistake, you know what I always think of? Everybody makes mistakes. Other people probably make just as many mistakes as I do. What is the difference if your teacher tells you in front of everyone?

Billie: The teacher corrected my mistakes after I worked so hard, and she didn't even say anything to this boy who didn't even do the work.

Dr. A.: He didn't even do his work? So he didn't even make mistakes! Your mistakes were better than what he did because to make mistakes is better than not doing the work.

Billie: But since he's not doing his work, he'll hear the teacher correct me, and then he'll get a better grade.

Dr. A.: I see. You're worried that he's gonna learn from your mistakes.

Billie: Yeah.

Dr. A.: You know, that's a good idea you have there. Somebody else can learn from your mistakes or from feedback that you get from somebody else. Does that give you any ideas about what you can learn from somebody else?

Billie: Yes! (*with a "aha" exuberance*)

Dr. A.: You can learn not only from your own mistakes but from somebody else's! If feedback tells you how you're doing, then can anyone tell me why it's important to know how you're doing? [No response from the children, who sit in a trance-like state.]

Nodal Point Discussion

Dr. A. had just done a combination of things that programmed the children to heightened suggestibility. One was the abrupt pattern disruption from the previous topic, which leaves the child hooked on the newly acquired insight before resistances or objections can develop. Another was the imbedded messages of "Feedback tells you how you're doing" and "It's important to know how you're doing." Another was the trance-derivational rhetorical question in which those messages were imbedded. The response of the children was a trance-like mental search for the answer, with slowing of motor activity and craving for an answer. At such times they are more suggestible, open to changes of attitude, and able to learn. It is a good time for a mini-lecture:

Dr. A.: If you keep track of how you're doing, you'll be making a big step forward for your emotional health. Feedback will kind of help you balance things out. One of the things I have seen happen to a lot of kids is when they are having a good day, they get carried away; then when something goes wrong, they get down in the dumps and think it's always going to be this way. Well, one of the things I learned from kids is that when things are going really well, remember that something can go wrong. Then if something does go wrong, it won't be so bad; you'll know this is what you expected. When things are going bad you can remember two things: how it was when it was going well and tomorrow may be a better day. What you do is kind of balance things out. When you're on a peak, pull yourself down, and when you're down, pull yourself up by thinking of how it was when it was better.

Dr. E.: I just wanted to ask if any of you kids have ever kept a diary? [Some of the children raise their hands.] Well, this is a way of getting feedback for yourself. Some people write down the good and bad things that happen each day. If you're having a bad day, you can read back through your diary to remember how it feels to have a good day.

Dr. A.: You can also look on the star charts to remind yourself of the good days and bad days, too.

Now let us return to the nodal point and see what happened on a different day with some of the same children with a similar question from Dr. A. On this occasion, the children did not look as trance-like and receptive but seemed more oriented to active participation:

Dr. A: Why is it important to know how you're doing? [There is no verbal response from the children, but some looked on the verge of speaking.] Come on, take a guess, Cindy?

Cindy: (*meekly*) So you can do it again? (*sounds uncertain*)

Dr. A.:   Right! Here is a good example of needing positive feedback—good feedback. Cindy answered right but didn't seem to know it. If I hadn't told her she was right, she would not have known. Not only is it important to have positive feedback but also negative feedback about things you did wrong. Why do you think negative feedback is good?

Howie: So you know what you did wrong.

Dr. A.:   OK. Good. (*looking around the room for some more answers*)

Kurt: So you can correct it.

Dr. A.:   You all three are right. If you know what you did right, you can do it again, and if you know what you did wrong, you can improve it. You can make changes to make it better.

On yet a third occasion, Kurt offered a colorful description of negative feedback:

Kurt: Feedback is when you hit someone over the head or when a big person looks at you in a funny way.

Dr. A.:   That's one kind of feedback. When you're about to do something wrong, parents let you know by a funny glare. Feedback means clues you get from other people. The way you get better is getting feedback from other people. Mrs. S. gives you feedback every week. What kind of feedback does Mrs. S. give you?

Billie: She tells us how we did in group.

Dr. E.:   What kinds of things does she tell you about?

Kurt: If we kept our hands to ourselves.

Tom: If we listened or asked permission.

Rick: If we paid attention to directions.

Paul: If we followed directions or stayed with the group.

Dr. E.:   That's very good. You all remembered what Mrs. S. gives you feed-back on. What I just said is feedback, too. Mrs. S. is giving you clues about your behavior. How does she give it to you?

Billie: With the star charts.

Dr. A.:   That's right. Mrs. S. gives you feedback about your behavior with the star chart. Do you think somebody would stop trying if they didn't have the star chart? [No verbal response.] Why would a kid not be interested in doing good if he didn't get stars? [No response; the children look baffled.]

Dr. A.:   In a situation where you don't get stars or a reward what would keep a kid going?

Mrs. F.:   You can get satisfaction knowing yourself that you can do it. It's kind of like a chart inside your head. As you grow up, you can make charts inside your head.

Dr. E.:   That's right. In the beginning, when you first learn to keep tabs on your behavior you need a chart (*to the parents*), something tan-gible, like Mrs. S. has done.

Dr. A.:   (*to the children*) When do you think you can get an inside chart, like grown-ups have? [The children look bewildered, and Dr. A. turns to the parents.] I think the kids still need outside charts.

A natural experiment demonstrated that the children did still need out-side charts. For several weeks, the routine of showing the star charts visually and verbally was neglected because of time pressure. By the third week, the children's group behavior had deteriorated to baseline. When star chart show and tell was restarted, group behavior dramatically improved in one week. One test ordinarily used to tell if a child is ready to graduate from the group is whether the child can go several weeks without group feedback (that is, suc-cessfully stretch the frequency of group attendance to two or three weeks instead of weekly).

17
Anger: The Inevitable Challenge

One of the lasting treasures a parent can give to a child is freedom of expression: freedom to express all feelings constructively, to deal comfortably with both positive and negative feelings. In many instances, this is not accomplished. It is particularly difficult for behavior-disordered children to learn because of their impulsiveness, tendency to action before verbalization, and parental fatigue.

When the foundations of positive, healthy, parent-child interactions are first cast, the child's way of expressing anger may be an annoyance to the parent. Parents often erroneously believe that feelings and actions are the same. They typically equate the child's way of expressing anger (the action or behavior) with the feeling (internal state) of anger and communicate to the child that one should not get angry. The belief is, "If he doesn't get angry, he won't behave this way." They overlook the fact that feelings cannot be controlled as readily as actions can. Adults need to define an attainable standard for the child. A five-year-old child, for example, cannot help feeling anger but can learn to refrain from hitting or punching.

What options do parents have in helping their children learn to deal with positive and negative feelings? Let's consider four options and their consequences:

1. Teach children to keep feelings bottled up inside and express none of them. Even if achieved, this could result in a constricted child or, more likely, in an eventual explosion.
2. Teach children to express only the positive feelings and none of the negative ones. The benefit is momentary positive parent-child interaction but at great cost: repression of negative feelings, resulting in later mental disorders.
3. Pay lip-service to letting the child express all feelings but provide subtle aversive consequences for expression of certain feelings This places the child in a double bind, with all the risks that it entails.
4. Teach children to express both positive and negative feelings but within

reasonable guidelines as to the manner, time, and place. Children are free to express feelings, such as anger, but are limited to means that are tolerable to both parent and child.

There are two possibilities for establishing the guidelines for expression: through unilateral decision by the parents or through mutual discussion and negotiation between parent and child. The first approach may be more appropriate with a younger child and the second approach with an older child.

In the first transcript excerpt, we explain to parents and children the principle of the safety valve and the necessity for letting off steam before the pressure builds up to an explosion. The second excerpt is an unusual example of a parent who is uncomfortable with his daughter's silent reaction to anger and would give anything for either a safety valve or an explosion.

Mrs. E.:   Recently I've sensed that something is wrong with Kurt. I don't know whether he's having some problems in school (haven't got any notes from the teacher) or what he's frustrated about. But every time he doesn't get his way at home, he goes into a temper tantrum like you've never seen: screaming and yelling, getting down on the floor, kicking his legs. It's so loud that it's embarrassing. The whole neighborhood can hear him. They probably think I'm beating him. I just wish I knew what was bothering him.

Dr. A.:   (*empathically nodding to Mrs. E.*) Well, one thing you can feel good about is: when a kid lets it out at home, I know he has a good home. He feels safe letting it out at home. They couldn't get away with it at school or with friends. It's a way of coping, but there is a limit as to what we can take. We need to set limits on it.

Dr. E.:   The children that we worry about the most are the ones that don't let it out at all. How do some of the others deal with anger?

Mrs. P.:   Neal gets into the same thing. I just tell him I don't want to have any part of him until he calms down. I tell him he can scream and yell all he wants, but I won't talk to him until he calms down. He blows up, and then it takes about fifteen minutes for him to calm down.

Dr. E.:   One thing that you mentioned that I like is that you talk to him after he calms down. That's good because things can be said in anger that we don't mean.

Dr. A.:   One technique that I like is actually asking a child how they would like to express anger. If you are dissatisfied with how negative feelings are being expressed in your family, decide with your child how anger is to be expressed. What you want to avoid is the volcanic eruption. This happens when parents close off all avenues of expression. Anger or certain feelings never get expressed because the child does not think to choose another means of expressing anger. When they don't like how certain feelings are being expressed, what parents can do is close off all other avenues and give permission to the one they want. Some parents close off all avenues, and children need at least one way, a safety valve. [Parents nod.]

Dr. E.:   On the inpatient unit when kids get angry, they like to get destructive. We give them old phone books to tear up. At home, kids, with the parents' permission, may decide to dig a hole outside, punch a bag, make something, or run around the block. Adults, too, find ways of releasing tension in a constructive way. They may clean house, work in the garden, or jog. [Parents nod understandingly.]

Dr. A.:   One important point is that adults can delay their release of tension, but a child has trouble waiting. If you set up a system that requires too long a delay, where they have no means of immediate expression, you are closing off the valves.

Dr. E.:   One thing I see happening a lot with parents is that they have a hard time adjusting to anger directed at them.

Mrs. E.:   Yes, I had that with my oldest daughter, Sally. All she had to say was, "I hate you, Mom"—like when I said "no" to her—and it was an immediate guilt trip. I would give in to her because I was so worried about my relationship with her. I guess I was just insecure and didn't have enough confidence in what I was doing.

Once I realized that her outbursts were momentary forms of release, I handled it better. I knew she didn't mean what she said. I just let her calm down. It took me a long time to understand this.

Dr. A.:   (*to the children after they returned from their separate group*) Today we were talking about ways of getting anger out. What can someone do so they don't do something wrong or something they don't mean to? We don't like being angry or nasty, but we have to get rid of the anger. Some people keep it inside, and others put it off until after work or school. Many times kids feel like they have to let it out right now. What about you kids? How do you feel? What if you kids want to play a game, and another kid didn't want to?

Billie: Well, I would go along with his and play mine later.

Dr. A.:   It doesn't always work that way for most kids. Some kids get angry and have to let it out right now. What about you, Kurt?

Neal: I would scream and yell. [Kurt laughs.]

Kurt: (*sarcastically*) I would hit a punching bag.

Dr. A.:   That's a good idea. Sometimes it works to plan what to do with your anger. Parents can decide with you how you get your anger out in your own family. How do some of the others get your anger out?

Sandra: I yell at her.

Paul: I'm patient.

Dr. A.:   Maybe you kids can ask your moms what way she would like you to get anger out. In fact, for next week's assignment, you can work it out with both Mom and Dad.

This unilateral assignment by the therapist differs from the usual practice of having the child pick an assignment with help from the parents. Child-picked assignments customarily are carried out successfully, but unilateral assignment by the therapist carries more risk of the assignment's not being done. How would you handle the following situation next week?

1. Parent or child or both could forget to carry out assignment: You could discover reasons why the assignment was not done. First, ask the child to say what the assignment was. If the child still forgets, ask the mother to repeat it. If the child can repeat it, acknowledge the answer, and ask the mother if that is how she understood it. Then ask what stopped the accomplishment. Restate the procedure of doing assignments weekly and the routine of telling the group how you did the following week. It is possible mother and child did not understand this routine. Help mother and child renegotiate the homework assignment now and make a commitment to it.

2. Perhaps the assignment was not done because the parents believe that

the child has no right to be angry. The child should be loyal and not complain. Options for answering include asking the mother what she means by "right." State that everyone has feelings. Quote theologians and moralists that feelings are not morally good or bad; they happen as part of our biological nature. Only action and decision can be morally bad. We cannot control what we feel, but we can control how we express feelings. Present an analogy to the mother, such as how she feels when the price of beef doubles yet her budget is the same. The choice is not whether to have feelings but what to do with them.

3. A third possibility is that the child has used Dr. A. as an excuse to act out anger destructively or manipulatively: "Dr. A. said I have to let anger out somehow if I didn't want to do what you said, and this is how I'm doing it." The most logical response here is to remind the child that the assignment was to find out the parent's wishes about how to express anger. The parents can be assured in front of the child that they do not need to accept the child's manipulation of the instruction.

Passive-Aggressive Anger

After listening to other parents, Mr. V., Billie's father, candidly divulged his feelings of frustration regarding how Billie expressed her anger and his ineffectiveness in dealing with it. As. Mr. V. talked, it appeared that the deterioration in their relationship was partly due to his superficial acceptance, which might be summarized thus: "If I am to be a good parent, I must accept the way she acts. I must accept her the way she is. There's nothing I can do; this is the way it is."

Mr. V.: This may seem kind of silly for grown-ups to worry about this, but, well, Pat, Billie's younger sister, is emotional. She'll come right out and say if she's mad like Sarah or if she's mad, she'll say, "You're unfair, you're on my back." She'll throw a temper tantrum, and we'll say, "Pat, go to your room." She'll come down from her room in five minutes and say, "I'm sorry I did what I did." She's different from Billie—just very spontaneous. You know exactly how she feels. We don't mind her getting mad. Billie, on the other hand, holds it in. I'd rather Billie explode once in a while.

Dr. E.: It seems like it's easier for you to deal with explicit rather than implicit feelings. It sounds like, too, that you're a little angry at Billie's passive-aggressive behavior. Once you recognize your own feelings about this, you can better deal with it. You may channel

Billie's expression of anger into something more adaptive or comfortable to you.

Mr. V.: Yes, I can deal with direct feelings better. I'll know exactly what's wrong that way. There is no pretense. With Billie, I feel there is a pretense.

Dr. E.: Rather than thinking of it as a pretense, I think it is a method Billie's discovered to deal with her anger. She deals with it in a passive way. Unfortunately, this type of behavior is effective in eliciting anger in parents, which is probably her aim: to rebel or defy. Perhaps Billie needs to be confronted with this. Then maybe she would begin to express her anger in more direct ways.

Mr. V.: I guess I didn't realize that this was what you call passive-aggressive behavior. I thought she was just putting on a pretense. I still don't know what to do about it.

Dr. E.: You can discuss with her the various ways people let their anger out, such as running around the block, punching a bag, taking a walk, digging a hole, pounding wood, a walk, etc., and ask her which one she would like to try. As a parent you can also model some of these.

Mr. V.: I guess I shouldn't expect her to be like her sister, Pat. [Three cheers for Mr. V.]

Rolling with the Punches

Below are hypothetical examples illustrating therapeutic handling of different responses at nodal points (crucial branches or forks in the discussion). They were devised to demonstrate how a discussion on anger can vary in content, logic, or emotional tone depending on the child's or parents' responses to the therapeutic exploration:

Dr. E.: (*to the children*) Today we were talking about ways of getting anger out, how kids get their anger out. Maybe you kids can tell me what people do and not do when they get angry. Can any of you kids tell me what people do and what they don't do when they get angry? [Puzzled looks.] Some kids scream and yell; some run
Nodal around; other kids go to their room. (*looking at Billie*) [Let's see
point 1 how Billie answers and what response suits her answer.]

Billie: Go to your room when you get angry?

Dr. E.:   I wonder if anybody knows that you're angry when you go to your room?

Billie: (*timidly*) I think so, yes.

Dr. E.:   (*looking at Mr. V.*) Maybe we could check with your dad to make sure he knows.

Mr. V.:   Well, to tell you the truth, I never knew, Billie; I had no idea you were angry. I thought you were playing some kind of game or putting on some pretense, acting as if you didn't care.

Dr. E.:   Billie, it's OK to feel angry at your parents, but maybe you could think of a more direct way of showing your anger or getting it out. [Billie shrugs.] If you can't think of anything at the moment, maybe you could ask your dad. Why don't you go ahead and ask him. Maybe he has some good ideas [Billie looks at her dad.]

Mr. V.:   Billie, maybe you could say, "I'm angry, Dad, or I'm mad at you," and then go to your room. What do you think of that? [Billie nods.]

Dr. E.:   I think that's good, but don't forget to discuss the problem afterward. Could both of you agree to work on this for next week's assignment?

Mr. V.
and Billie: (*smiling at each other*) Yes.

Dr. E.:   Good, We'll be looking forward to seeing how you do.

Now let us return to nodal point 1 and see how other children respond and an alternate development:

Dr. E.:   Can any of you kids tell me what people do and not do when they get angry?

Neal: I'd scream and yell.

Robert: I don't say anything.

Dr. E.:   (*to Robert*) You don't say anything? You mean you keep it a secret?

Robert: I guess.

Dr. E.:   Do you think you can really keep your parents from knowing you're angry?

Robert: Yep.

Dr. E.:   Wonder why someone would want to keep it a secret? Robert, maybe you can tell us why someone would keep it a secret? [Robert **Nodal** looks confused.] Maybe some of the other kids have some ideas **point 2** why someone would keep it a secret when they are angry? Can anyone tell me? (*looking around to all the children*)

Billie: Maybe they are afraid to tell their parents they are angry.

Dr. E.:   That's a good idea! Maybe somebody's afraid to tell their parents. Why do you think somebody would be afraid to tell their parents they are angry?

Billie: Maybe if they tell, they're afraid they'll get punished.

Dr. E.:   I see; somebody might worry that they would get punished. Robert, did you ever worry that you would get punished if you told your mother you were angry?

Robert: Yes.

Dr. E.:   You did! Maybe you should check with your mom about that. Maybe you can ask her right now if she would punish you if you told her you were angry. [Note the technique of questioning his mom in front of the group. Even if she were the type of parent who preferred keeping feelings bottled up, the peer pressure is great enough to elicit an appropriate answer, and the principle of cognitive dissonance might persuade her to follow her own answer. [Robert looks at his mother, Mrs. A., but doesn't have enough courage to ask her.]

Mrs. A.:   Well, of course, I wouldn't punish you, honey. I would like very much for you to tell me when you're angry.

Dr. E.:   Robert, did you hear that! Your mom said she wouldn't punish you. She would like you to tell her that you are angry. [Robert shakes head.] No! Well, instead of keeping it a secret, Robert, you have to pick another way of showing your anger. Maybe some of the other kids can help you out?

Kurt: You can run around the block.

Tom: You can make something or punch a bag!

Dr. E.:   Both of those are good ideas. Robert, why don't you pick one, as long as your mother will agree on it, too. Which one do you want to pick?

Robert: I'll punch a bag.

Dr. E.:   OK, Robert. Make sure its OK with your mom. [Mrs. A. nods.] Well, we'll see how you do this week. You can report to us next time.

Let us return to nodal point 2 and see how a different reason for keeping anger a secret is handled:

Dr. E.:   Oh. I wonder why a kid would keep it a secret?

Sarah: Cuz may be they'd be afraid of hurting their parents' feelings.

Dr. E.:   That's one reason. Which way do you think would hurt the parents' feelings more: keeping it a secret or telling them how you feel even if it's not nice? [Sarah looks confused.] Maybe one of the adults can help us out.

Mrs. E.:   I guess keeping it a secret.

Dr. E.:   That's what I think, too. Why is that?

Mrs. E.:   Because if they keep it a secret, you don't know exactly what's wrong and it hurts to see your child upset.

Dr. E.:   (*to the children*) They wouldn't know what's the matter, and parents get hurt easily when they don't know what's the matter with their kid. Can anyone else tell me why a kid would keep their anger a secret? Does anyone else have any ideas?

Kurt: (*shrewdly*) Cuz you can really get to your parents then!

Dr. E.:   That's like cutting off your nose to spite your face. Hurting your-self to hurt your parents. I bet everyone has done that once. [Everyone nods.] Kurt, I think I might tell you that you would get more from your parents if you cooperated with them. One of the things you can do is ask your mom how she would like you to show your anger. Could you do that?

Kurt: (*halfheartedly*) All right. [He turns to his mother and asks her.]

18
Separation

One thing that therapy and child rearing have in common is the pervasive inevitability of eventual separation. The threat and promise of separation color all transactions and tempt the participants to denial, worry, or counterphobic escape. Ambivalent hope pervades all. The successful parent loses a child (but gains a friend); the successful child loses a parent (but gains a friend); the successful therapist loses a patient (but gains professional fulfillment); the successful patient loses a therapist (but gains health).

Therapy must deal from the beginning with termination–separation issues. It has even been said that successful termination is the main work of psychotherapy. Certainly, titrating appropriate levels of dependence, autonomy, and separation is one of the main tasks of the parent-child relationship.

Life brings many reminders of the ultimate separation. Among these are moves, changes of school, termination of therapy, and loss of friends. This chapter deals with only two of these.

A Moving Experience

Mrs. E., Craig's mother, brought up her concern about the difficulty her son was having since their move from another city:

Mrs. E.: He's a bright boy, but he didn't want to move, and now his behavior problems are interfering with his learning in school. I won't play his little games. He has set fires because he wants to move back to Gotham City. It's an attack on me. He needs help, and he's painted himself in a corner now. He's scared because he knows I've reached the end of my rope.

Think how you would respond to the issues Mrs. E. ventilated about. Would it be more effective to respond to the general issue of the move or these specific issues: Craig's learning problem, Craig's fire-setting behavior, the frustration his mother feels, an explanation of Craig's hostility to his mother, or his mother's assumption of warlike relationship with her son. Each of these issues is important enough to deserve exploration if it were not competing for time with other important issues. This mother eventually needed some individual guidance, especially to deal with the last issue. The choice at this point needed to be based on what would be best for the whole group, as well as Mrs. E. Commenting on the move and the issue of separation would be more conducive to the group process because this is a universal problem that the other parents easily identify with.

Dr. A.:   One issue that you just brought up, all of which were important, is the move. Has anyone else had trouble with a move?

Mr. B.:   In our case, the move worked to Bob's advantage. He would have had to repeat the first grade and was worried about what his friends would think. Now that we moved, Bob has had a fresh start, and the problem resolved itself.

Mr. C.:   We didn't have any problems with a move, either. Although we moved into a new school district, we didn't move out of town, so he [Dan] still gets to see his old friends.

Mrs. E. is looking more frustrated; no one has provided the support she needs. Dr. A. is also feeling frustrated because the support he expected the other parents to offer was not forthcoming. In retrospect, perhaps he should have set the stage or otherwise hinted at the kind of response he wanted from the other parents by providing the following explanation before asking for the other parents' input, but he figured better late than never, and was able to salvage the situation:

Dr. A.:   In many instances when the move occurs, it is the parents that are really the ones that are happy with the move. Perhaps they are looking forward to the new house or promotion. But with kids, an adjustment period is required. They don't see the advantages of the changes, and they like the stability and security of the old. It's like being separated from a loved one. [All the parents nod, including Mrs. E.]

Dr. A. had the opportunity to bring up the issue of separation in the combined parent-child segment when it was time to announce to the group that he would not be present the following week.

Dr. A.:   I just wanted to mention that I will not be here next week. I will be away, but the rest of the staff will be here. Has anyone had the experience of having to leave someone or someone leaving you, as in death or divorce? [All the children nod.] What age do you think you have to get to be so that it won't bother you?

Heidi: Twenty!

Dr. A.:   I'll have to agree with you that by age twenty it's easier to handle because by that age you have learned to deal with separation.

Mrs. J.:   Is there an age? I wouldn't think there would be?

Dr. A.:   Yes, you're right. There's no age, but through the years and as you get older, you learn to get better at it. What can you do to get better at it—like a kid who leaves the group—so it will help you next time somebody leaves you or you have to leave?

Tom: I don't know. What can you do?

Dr. A.:   Tom, I like the way you just asked when you didn't know something. If you ask questions when you don't know something, it will be a big help in life! Now as far as what you can do, does anyone have any ideas? [The other children are at a loss for words.]

Dr. E.:   You can discuss your worry or concern with somebody close to you: parents, sisters and brothers, or other relatives, or a close friend.

Dr. A.:   OK. Is there anything else? [The group is intently thinking.] Well, you can use your memory. As long as you can remember a person, are they really gone? They're not completely gone are they? [Several adults nod; the children look surprised as they notice the adults' agreement.] As long as you can remember the good times, then that person will be alive to you.

Paul: If you leave the group or move, you can keep contact after a person's gone.

Dr. A.:   That's right! You can call them, go see them, take pictures of them to look at after they are gone, or talk to them by phone.

In the preceding vignette, Dr. A. hinted that the experience of leaving the group could be a rehearsal for other separations, a learning experience, through which one can learn to separate more adaptively. In the following vignette, one of the parents picked up on this hint.

Giving the Child Some Control

In the parents' group, Mrs. A., Robert's mother, shared her concern about how one makes the decision to quit the group. The reason they had started coming to the group was her son's behavior problems in school. Although Robert was doing fine now, Mrs. A. still felt worried because of Robert's adverse reaction to loss, for example, when a friend leaves the house. In the parents' group, we assured Mrs. A. that we too had noticed Robert's progress and implied permission to quit the group.

She was advised that it was desirable for the youngster to have some choice in the timing of group termination, which would shore up his feeling of control and reinforce him for his good behavior, as well as soften any separation pains he might feel. An additional advantage is giving the child a choice to prevent a situation that we have seen occasionally, in which a child deliberately misbehaves in order to force return to the group after a parental decision to terminate. Mrs. A. agreed with the idea of giving Robert some choice, and it seemed an appropriate group ceremony when the children rejoined the parents:

Dr. A.: One of the things that was mentioned in the parents' group was about quitting the group. Maybe I should mention to the others who we are talking about. Robert and his mother are thinking about stopping the group since Robert has made so much progress on what he came in for. (*to Robert*) Do you want to come back two or three times, or do you want to quit now? [Robert is hesitant.] You know some kids have a hard time saying they want to quit because they are afraid we'll be hurt and we won't let them come back if they want to. Do you feel like that? [Robert, pensive and ambivalent, nods.] Robert, you can come back any time you want to. We won't be mad. We're used to it. Also, if things are getting rough, will you tell us? You may want to come back. Maybe your mother can tell us. [Robert, looking relieved, exchanges smiles with both mother and Dr. A. and states that he is ready to stop. He and the other children exchange farewells.]

19
Relatives

Child rearing is one of the favorite targets of kibbitzing. Everyone kibbitzes: neighbors, talk show guests and hosts, columnists, various professionals, the authors of this book. The most entitled kibbitzers of all are grandparents and other relatives. Grandparents feel especially entitled when something has gone wrong with the child. Therefore, parents of any handicapped child and especially parents of a behavior-disordered child have added to their other frustrations the burden of free advice and criticism from kibbitzers who are confident that they could handle the child better and who feel virtuous about protecting the child from the parents' ineptness.

If a parent already tends to feel guilty, as is often the case, the kibbitzers enthusiastically confirm the judgment. If the parents feel overprotective, the kibbitzers reinforce or vie to be more protective. If the parent feels rejection toward the child, the added harassment provides more justification for the rejection. Perhaps the rejection is even embellished with the accusation that the child's problem is a punishment for the sin of a parent.

When grandparents have attended the group, their presence has been helpful in improving grandparent-parent relations. When a grandparent is living with the family, it is useful to invite the grandparents along with the parents, unless they object (they never have objected in our experience). Whether grandparents are present in body or not in the group, their presence in spirit is often felt.

There are various ways to begin the parent separate group. One way is to pick up a problem (or sometimes a bit of good news) that cropped up during the initial combined parent-child group. On this occasion Neal P., who had been previously enthusiastic and successful with his assignments, reported a week of zero success. Since zero success is unusual, it should not be ignored. One of the best ways to maintain a positive, hopeful attitude in the group is to demonstrate fearlessness in confronting any problems or discouragements as they occur. In this vignette Dr. E. models a problem-solving attitude toward Neal's bad report.

Dr. E.:   (*to Mrs. P.*) It seems as if Neal must have had a bad week. He did not follow through with his assignment. What do you think happened?

Mrs. P.: We had a bad week. You're right. Neal yells at his grandmother, who lives with us, and I yelled at Neal for yelling at his grandmother. Then his grandmother and I got into it, and by then Neal just walked away.

It was obvious that Neal had projected some conflict of his own onto his grandmother and mother; he made it their fight, not his. It would be tempting to broach that interpretation at this point. Mrs. P. would probably have seen such an interpretation as a brilliant revelation, and it might have made her think twice about jumping into the grandmother-grandchild fray in the future. If such an interpretation were made, a good way to do it might be: "It must be very frustrating to you to be fighting his battles for him with grandmother" or "How often does he get you to fight with grandmother for him?" However, Dr. A. and Dr. E. chose to pursue a less flashy, less interpretive course:

Dr. E.:   Does this happen frequently, that Neal yells at his grandmother?

Mrs. P.: Yes, all the time, and he gets away with bloody murder.

Dr. A.:   Does it seem to bother Grandmother that Neal yells at her? [Dr. A. is wondering if Mrs. P. is taking responsibility for something that is not really a problem.]

Mrs. P.: I'm not sure, but she and I get into it. She makes me feel bad for yelling at Neal, and she seems to be protecting him.

Dr. E.:   How do some of the others handle overprotective grandparents? How much should grandparents interfere? Should they discipline the children?

Mrs. V.: Well, we have my mother living with us, and she just isn't the type to take assertion. She instead comes to me and tells me what happened. I have to make up the rules and tell her, for example, that Ted is not allowed to leave the yard. If he does something wrong, then she tells me about it, and then I have to deal with it.

Dr. E.:   Are you comfortable with the way things are going with that?

Mrs. V.: Yes, I am.

Dr. E.:   You don't expect grandmother to deal with it?

Mrs. P.:   Well, I tell my mother to just spank him real hard if he deserves it, and she won't do it. Then I get mad at her. She did it to me, so why shouldn't she do it to him, like he was her own son?

Mrs. F.:   It seems like it's a real problem having grandparents around. We don't have our relatives around, and I had always thought that Howie and the rest of the family were really missing out, but now I don't know . . .

Mrs. F. changes the topic to a problem with Howie's not letting her know where he went after school. In retrospect, Dr. E. wishes she had reached some closure on the topic of relatives before pursuing Mrs. F.'s concern. It could have been done like this:

Dr. E.:   Before pursuing that, Mrs. F., I'd like to tie up a few loose ends. Relatives can be a problem at times. It's not that they don't mean well; it's just that dealing with your child's handicap is as difficult for them as it is for you. As a result, they often say or do things that are not helpful. They need to learn from you how to handle the situation. Just as you often feel up, down, guilty, or protective about your child, they do, too.

After the children returned, the discussion was reintroduced:

Dr. A.:   One of the things that we talked about with your parents, that I think you might find interesting is grandparents! What do you kids think about grandparents?

Howie: They are your mother's and father's parents.

Dr. A.:   Right! What about discipline? Do you think grandparents should discipline?

Howie: It depends on their health. If they are real old, they might get sick.

Dr. A.:   What if they were healthy?

Howie: If they were healthy, I think they should do the punishment.

Dr. E.:   Who should decide on the punishment: the kids, the parents, or the grandparents?

Ted: Well, I think the kids should decide with the parents. [This is an interesting comment by Ted since his parents had taken a rigid view on this subject, deciding that they should be the ones to choose a punishment.]

Harley: I think the parents should decide because kids would be too easy on themselves.

Dr. A.:   That's possible. How many of you think the parents should decide? [All the children raise their hands.] Then you don't think the grandparents should decide?

Howie: No, just the parents.

Ted: Just the parents. [Neal and Harley nod.]

Dr. A.:   Sounds like you all think the parents should be boss. [The children nod.]

Not all kibbitzing by relatives is bad. One example is an aunt who came to group with a four-year-old boy and his mentally retarded mother, supported both of them in making use of the group for behavioral management, and eventually took both of them into her home when the mother was not able to manage by herself. Another example is a grandmother who came to the group and garnered assistance from other group members in confronting the child's mother with the fact that she was undervaluing herself and depriving herself too much in order to cater to the child's whims. A third example is a grandfather who attended the group regularly with his grandson, whose divorced mother had to work during group hours; he maintained communication between the boy's mother and the group staff.

20
Timing, Pacing, and Finesse in Limit Setting

Timing and pacing, relatively neglected topics, must be considered in any child management approach, if for no other reason than that the managee is a child for only a limited time. This fact and some of its ramifications are elaborated in the first section of this chapter on procrastination, appeasement, escalation, and inflation. The issue of pacing is more specifically addressed in the second section on the countdown. The third section explores the relationship of timing, options, finesse in limits and punishment, and induction of self-limits. The first section shows the group leaders in a very active (perhaps too active), directive role, with minisermons of advice; the third section shows a more facilitative role.

Inflation and Escalation

Penny's mother, Mrs. T., after several weeks of therapy, commiserates and serves as consultant to another parent:

Mrs. T.: Children need to know what the rules are. Penny, when we first started, was a terror. I couldn't get her to do nothing. Since I work full time, I wanted everyone in the house to share the chores. I made a rule that everyone had to clean house. No matter how I screamed and yelled, she never did it. We'd end up in huge battles, but she always got her way. She'd upset me so much saying, "I hate you, you're a witch," that I'd just give up. It was a lot easier after a long day. After coming here, I found out it's sort of like training a dog. You have to train them when they're little; you can teach them, then. When they get older, you might as well forget it. Let them think you're a villain!

Dr. E.: You really zeroed in on an important point, Mrs. T. Things may get worse before they get better. Maybe when she's older one day, she'll appreciate what you are trying to do now. But don't expect her to tell you that now.

Dr. A.: You seem to have seen through the appeasement or procrastination fallacy. With a three-year-old, you may give in to a temper tantrum because it seems so harmless or even cute, or you feel sorry for the poor frustrated kid, and it seems a small price to keep her happy or to keep peace. And you might figure she'll outgrow it and be more reasonable to deal with later. But as long as she can get everything she wants by such demands, there is no reason to outgrow them. In behavior modification terms, the demands and tantrums are reinforced. With a five-year-old, the tantrum may be worse and harder to resist or endure, so you still give in. With an eight-year-old, it becomes even more of a problem. She may threaten to hurt herself, so you give in. A fifteen-year-old may try to threaten you with a drug overdose. What parents with young children don't realize is that if they don't limit it, it keeps getting worse, not better.

Dr. E.: Yes. It's unlikely that they will just grow out of it as long as they got what they want by it.

Dr. A.: It's a lot harder to set limits on a ten-year-old than it is to set limits on a three-year-old, but it will be even harder at age fifteen if you don't start now.

Dr. E.: (*to Mrs. T.*) It seems that you have begun to realize this.

Mrs. T.: The hardest thing of all is to realize what's happening, but most of all it is the time, patience, and persistence it takes.

Dr. E.: Are you saying that you sometimes feel tired of it all?

Mrs. T.: (*sounding a little depressed*) Yes, I do. I just wish I had done all these things earlier so it wouldn't be so hard now.

Dr. E.: I guess that's true. We can all look back and realize what we should have done. But feel good that you know now and she has made some progress with your efforts. If you hadn't started now, she may have become uncontrollable at fifteen.

Mr. Q.: The thing that bothers me is that I just don't have the heart to say "no" to things he wants that I know he shouldn't have.

Dr. E.: Why not?

Mr. Q.: Well, I guess . . . Oh, I don't know. Maybe it's because I didn't have much when I was a kid and I want to give him the best.

Dr. E.: It's typical for parents to want to give their children more than they've had. But there are limits. Decide what and when to give and give that freely, but no more, no matter what he does or how guilty he makes you feel.

Dr. A.: The price keeps going up. It escalates. You have to have it out now because when he's big, it will be harder [Mrs. T. nods as if to say "Believe it."], so you might as well have it out now. [Mr. Q. still looks uncomfortable and doubtful.]

Dr. E.: (*to Mr. Q.*) It seems that Kevin needs to learn that the world does not owe him or that you don't owe him. He must learn to take responsibility for his actions and earn privileges. [Mr. Q. nods.]

Mrs. T.: It's a funny thing. I didn't realize this before. But somehow kids like you a lot better if you do what we've been saying.

Dr. E.: They respect you more, too.

Dr. A.: Maybe you like yourself more too. [Mrs. T. nods.]

This vignette is presented partly as an example of advice overkill. The use of minilectures or sermonettes (motivating explanations of a problem) is a useful technique for parents' groups. It is also useful at times for a coleader to restate the other leader's point in different words or for the two leaders to dialogue (and demonstrate resolution of a problem or disagreement). The summation of all three leader activities in this case seems too much, however. In fairness to Dr. A. and Dr. E., the parents were interacting nonverbally, so that the process was not as leader lopsided as it appears in transcript. Nevertheless, this session's effectiveness could have been increased by one of the leaders playing devil's advocate for the resistant Mr. Q. to identify with and then allowing himself to be convinced gradually by the rest of the group.

The Countdown

Many children perpetually test their parent's rank and power. Parents of children are caught between a hard rock and soft spot. Although they may understand the necessity to establish themselves as boss and set firm limits to organize the children's disorientation and chaotic world and to help them learn to live with rules, a skill they will need all their lives, their feelings about the child's handicap often prevent them from taking such a hard line. Further, even when they decide to be firm, the child's inattentiveness and perceptual deficits may interfere with receiving the message of firmness. One way to establish the parent's confidence and control, to structure the limit setting, to channel the parent's frustration, and to focus the child's attention on the fact that a limit is being set is the countdown.

The countdown is a way for parents to communicate to their children their serious intent, their intent to apply an ultimate aversive consequence consistently if the countdown fails, and their intent to use a warning system first, the countdown, in hopes that the aversive consequence will not be necessary. We sometimes recommend to parents the following excerpt from *Parent's Survival Handbook* (pp. 14–15), which elaborates on instructions given orally in the parent's group:

The warning method we prefer is to **precede the primary zinger** (aversive consequence) **with a count of three.** This is especially effective when there is too much silliness or uproar to get the child's attention with a simple, firm command. The switch from ordinary words to numbers is an abrupt enough intrusion that it ordinarily attracts the child's attention, and clearly signals that something special is happening. Furthermore, it provides a very clear external cue to the child as to how much time he has to comply. It also provides some pacing and discipline for the parent, who may be tempted otherwise to issue one more repetitive warning instead of acting. Best of all, it is beautifully suited to be developed into a secondary zinger.

If consistently used and faithfully followed through on, the count to three will gradually evolve the quality of a secondary zinger. This phenomenon is well known in conditioning theory. When a neutral stimulus is always closely followed by another stimulus, it assumes some of the power of that other stimulus. If the count of three is always associated with a terrible consequence, the child will begin to fear the count of three almost as much as the consequence that it heralds. Thereupon he will feel anxious enough at the count of two that he will act quickly to prevent three. This, of course, is what you would like to have: some simple verbal means of letting the child know you mean business without having to resort to punishment or otherwise exert yourself unnecessarily. Further, the child's compliance, at the count of two, by relieving his anxiety, becomes rewarding or reinforcing of itself. (It is a good idea to add external reinforcement by thanking him for complying and allowing him to shift into a positive relationship with you.) Eventually, the count of two, as the harbinger of three, may take on the qualities of a tertiary zinger and be anxiously avoided by prompt, self-reinforcing compliance at the count of one. And the decisive, firm instruction preceding the count of one should eventually produce enough compliance to obviate even the count of one most of the time.

For this to occur, you will need to invest a little time and energy in the beginning to work on your pacing of the count and to follow through ruthlessly whenever the child by his sluggishness allows you to get to the count of three. To be most effective, the count should be **barked out clearly, crisply and inexorably,** with a pacing that gives the feeling of a lumbering steam roller that cannot be resisted, but which allows sufficient time to scramble out of its way. Tirades do not serve the purpose.

It is desirable to **restate the command** at the time of the countdown: "I said to stop throwing sand! One! . . . Two! . . . Three! . . ." Or alternately: "One! I said to stop throwing sand! Two! . . . Three!" If the child complies before 3, stop the count and thank him graciously. To be able to shift gears to a gracious gratitude, you must have started the count before you lose your cool. If you reach the count of three, terrible consequences must inevitably and quickly descend on the child like a bolt of avenging justice (short of brutality or child abuse, of course).

The **pacing** of the count is extremely important. Too rapid a count does not allow time for the child to comply, and you will arrive at three realizing you shouldn't have. Too slow a count may lull the child into believing you don't have the heart to carry through to the count of three. Approximately one or two seconds hesitation between numbers is about right. A little reflection will suggest that the most important interval of all is that between one and two, because we hope never to reach three. The pacing and tone of the two should leave the impression that three is almost on the way and there is no time to waste.

There will be times when you will not want to carry through after the count of three, either because you just don't feel up to it or because the problem does not seem worth the fuss (you should not have started the countdown in the first place if the issue was not worth the fuss). Remember that the countdown is a communication that you are serious, and it packs its wallop because it symbolizes what will follow if the child does not respond in time. This means that you should **only start the count when you are willing to finish it and follow through.** You should only start counting in situations where you would eventually uncork your primary zinger if you were not using the countdown. If you give into the temptation to use it as a bluff in other situations, you risk having the bluff called and finding yourself trapped in a dilemma of your own making. You will be forced either to punish against your better judgment or to sabotage the credibility of the countdown by backing off.

Eventually, of course, you will find that as the more serious behavior comes under control, you can gradually raise the standards and extend the countdown to less serious behavior, practically never reaching the count of three. This possibility can be realized only by taking the time, effort, and agony to establish the countdown initially.

(Reprinted from *Parents' Survival Handbook* by permission, LAMMP Publishing Co., Box 262, Sunbury, Ohio 43074.)

Handling Stale Misbehavior

Mrs. T.:	Somebody told me yesterday that last week David broke out some windows with a hammer and hit another boy with a rock. I don't know what to do when I hear about bad behavior so long afterwards. It doesn't seem to make much sense to whip him then, so I try to talk with him about it, but I'm not sure whether I'm doing the right thing. Maybe I'm letting him get away with something.
Dr. A.:	How do the others handle it when you hear about misbehavior long afterward?
Mrs. E.:	That's a tough one. I usually confront him with it. But I'm puzzled about what to do when he tells me about it himself. I don't want to punish him for telling me the truth, but I don't want him to think it's OK to do something wrong just because he tells me about it.
Dr. A.:	That sounds similar to Mrs. T.'s dilemma.
Mrs. C.:	I usually talk with him [Dan] about it and maybe try to get him to agree that it was a bad thing to do.
Dr. A.:	How about you, Mrs. M.?
Mrs. M.:	I hate that situation. One time I just told him how disappointed I was.
Dr. A.:	This does seem to be a very difficult situation to know what to do, because you don't want to let him feel he's getting away with something or condone it, but on the other hand you don't feel it makes much sense to drag up something out of the past that you have just found out about from somebody else. What are the various options you might have? One, of course, is to punish, as Mrs. T. considered. Another is to confront him, as Mrs. E. said. This could involve either scolding or explaining. What else? [no response] How about ignoring? Is that a possible option?
Several parents:	Yes . . . never thought of that . . . might be easier.

Dr. A.:   There are two ignoring options. You could ignore it with his knowing that you know, in which case he would always be waiting for the other shoe to drop, and the suspense might keep him on his good behavior, or you could ignore it secretly with his thinking you don't know in which case he might worry enough about you finding out to make him wish he hadn't done it (A kind of guilt enhancement).

Mrs. T.:   What if someone tells you in front of him and acts like they expect you to do something?

Dr. A.:   That kind of takes away your option of ignoring, doesn't it?

Mrs. T.:   Maybe then I could try sharing how I feel.

Mrs. E.:   And maybe you could have him make restitution.

Mrs T. began this session by addressing Dr. A. with a problem that she did not see a solution for. Dr. A.'s objectives in asking the others how they handled it were to establish that this was a shared concern so that everyone could feel some commitment to carrying on the discussion; to see if the parents could help each other with this situation; to avoid telling group members what they already knew; and to define the facilitator's role. As facilitator, it was appropriate to summarize at various points the material contributed by various members of the group and to supplement it with information they were not able to think of by themselves. Dr. A. modeled an approach of thinking about various options as preparation for deciding what could be done in a given situation. Eventually other parents picked up on this techniques. When Mrs. T. presented complicatons of her original problem and the leader dropped a hint about thinking of options by saying that this complication eliminated one of the options, two of the parents were able to come up with options that had not been eliminated.

After the children returned from their separate group, the discussion was reintroduced:

Dr. A.:   Today we were talking about something very important, something that you kids may be interested to know about and something maybe you can help figure out. One of the things the parents were talking about was when you kids do something wrong and then somebody else tells your mom or dad about it. Does that ever happen? [All of the children nod.] Darn those tattlers! [The children laugh.] One of the things parents mentioned was that they do not feel sure about how to handle it. Did you know your parents would ever worry about that? [All children look bewildered except Kurt.]

Kurt: That's a joke.

Dr. A.: What do you mean?

Kurt: Any time they get a chance to punish us, I bet they're glad.

Dr. A.: Let's see how some of the other kids feel. Do you think parents like to punish kids? Sarah? [Look pensive.] Neal? [Looks perplexed.] Penny? [Looks indifferent.]

Sarah: They have to because they're our parents.

Dr. E.: That's right, Sarah. They have to because it's their duty. I guess it's a funny way parents show you they care or that they love you. Penny, what do you think? Do you think parents like to punish their kids? [Penny shrugs.] Maybe some of the adults can tell us, then.

Mrs. T.: I wish these kids would realize that we hate to punish you kids, but sometimes you put us in the position where we have to: it's either you or me!

Mrs. E.: I just wish that they would realize it hurts us just as much.

Dr. A.: Did you kids realize that—that it hurts your parents just as much to punish you? [The children still look surprised.] Let me ask you this. What if you came and told your mom or dad about a week after you did something bad. What do you think your parents should do? Do you think your parents should punish you?

Kurt: That would be dumb! I wouldn't tell my mother.

Dr. A.: What about the rest of you? What do you think?

Sarah: If I told my mother, I would want her to be understanding.

Dr. A.:   Why do you think a kid would tell his parents he did something bad? If he kept it a secret like the way Kurt would want, his parents would never know. Right?

Penny: [Penny is the oldest in the group.] Well, I guess if somebody told their mom, they must've felt bad or something like that.

Dr. E.:   You mean maybe they felt guilty? Sometimes that's enough punishment, isn't it?

Penny: Maybe they could make it up. [Mrs. T., Penny's mother is surprised.]

Dr. A.:   We still haven't answered the question. Even if a kid tells their mom they did something bad, how many of you think they should make it up? [All hands raise except Kurt.]

Dr. E.:   Maybe you don't have to tell your mom every time you do something wrong. You can admit it to yourself. (*looking at Kurt*) One of the hardest things in life to learn is to say either to yourself or others, that you've made a mistake. Some adults have trouble with it, too. If you can learn to do it when you're young, then you'll really be at an advantage.

21
Punishment

Punishment is an interesting expression of parental love. One of the chief complaints by many parents is that their punishment efforts are not appreciated or rewarded. At least, they have not been able to detect enough results of punishment to justify this expenditure of energy and parental concern. Many of these parents at first appear punitive in their desperate attempt to get results. Others have not been consistent in applying limits or punishment because of their own ambivalence or conflicts about being the heavy. The parents' discomfort about the punishment arrangement is often shared by the children (who often see their parents as punitive), but in some instances they are unconcerned as well as unresponsive to punishment.

Although limit setting, punishment, and reward are different, they are intricately connected and cannot be discussed in isolation from each other. Limits that the child ignores often have to be enforced; punishment therefore often follows closely on limit setting. On the other hand prompt, early, clear and unequivocal limit setting, as well as rewarding the competing behavior, can often prevent the need for punishment. Therefore, even though limits were dealt with more extensively in the previous chapter and rewards were discussed in chapter 9, both occasionally come up in the clinical examples in this chapter.

We have found the following strategies helpful in dealing with the punishment issues that repeatedly crop up in multifamily group therapy:

1. Define the purpose of punishment.
2. Define what makes a punishment effective (to achieve the purpose, not to hurt the child or do justice).
3. Support parents in their obligation and right to set limits and punish in serious matters of safety, health or rights of others.
4. Help parents find alternate ways of preventing undesirable behavior, such as early limit setting, structuring the situation, and rewarding competing behaviors.
5. Help the child see parental limit setting and punishment as helpful rather than hostile.

6. Help the child see that punishment and limit setting are mandated by cultural norms above the parent, not merely parental whim.
7. Help the parents shoulder the psychological burden of being the heavy by instructing them in front of the child to be strict when such advice is indicated. In cases where parents are unable to limit or punish effectively because of their own residual conflicts and guilt, they may need permission and sometimes even need to have the guilt channeled into the service of being firm by defining the latter as a parental duty.

This chapter uses clinical excerpts from three sessions to illustrate the application of these strategies.

Negotiating from Strength

The I. family arrived a few minutes after the group split into separate parents' and children's sections. After listening to the other parents, Mr. I. brought up his dissatisfaction with the negotiating he always had to do with his son whenever he wanted to punish him. He indicated that it was his understanding they were supposed to negotiate over such things. This misunderstanding apparently related to an arrangement made about four months previously in which Mrs. I. and Manny were helped to negotiate an agreement whereby he would do certain chores and take care of certain responsibilities in exchange for her not nagging him about them ahead of time. She had been anticipating that he would not do them and she would start nagging him before he had a chance to do them. Then he would passive-aggress by not doing them.

As Mr. I. talked, it appeared that his main objection was not so much the negotiating but that this often resulted in a penalty that did not seem to him sufficiently large; justice was not done. When asked whether his top priority was to change Manny's behavior in a favorable direction or to see that an appropriate penalty is paid, he indicated that he thought the latter was the important thing, and any favorable change in behavior was merely a bonus. All the other parents in the group, including his own wife, indicated that they thought a favorable change in behavior was the main priority. One of the mothers said that she was not interested at all in seeing just retribution. Mrs. I. said that she thought just retribution was important but not important enough to sacrifice behavior improvement for.

In the middle of this discussion, the children returned from their separate activity. Ordinarily their return can be accepted at almost any point in the parents' discussion, because whatever topic the parents are talking about usually can be quickly adapted to the children's participation, with appropriate change in emphasis. On this particular occasion, it seemed important for Mr. I. to be able to hear the message from other parents and from the professionals that his priorities were misplaced. Since the children's presence would not permit that, Mrs. S. was asked to take the children to another room for about ten minutes and continue some of their activities. The parents then finished.

When the children returned again, the issues had been sufficiently clarified to adapt the topic to the children's participation:

Dr. A.: (*to the children*) The parents have been talking about something that is probably very important to you kids: punishment. One of the interesting things that came out is that they have the impression that you kids don't like punishment! [Laughter.] Is that right? (*directed to each of the children in turn, each of whom affirms a dislike of punishment*) Then why do you suppose they punish you? Do you think they enjoy it? [One child shakes his head; the others look baffled.] Maybe we should ask the parents about that. [Dr. A. goes around the room checking with parents, who unanimously state a dislike for needing to punish.] Well that's rather curious. You kids don't like to be punished, and your parents don't like to punish you. How come they do it? [The children look bewildered.] Maybe we should ask your parents.

Mr. I.: (*to Manny*) Because I want you to grow up to be a good citizen—like me. [Laughter.]

Dr. A.: (*to kids*) Who do you think should decide on the punishment: the kid being punished or the person giving the punishment?

Rick: The person giving the punishment.

Kurt: The person giving the punishment.

Dr. A.: Manny, how about you?

Manny: The person giving the punishment.

Dr. A.: That's right. The person giving the punishment makes the final decision about it. Of course, that person might ask the advice of the kid about what would be the best punishment or might give the kid the choice between two different punishments, but that's only if the adult decides that's the way he wants to do it. Does it do any good for the kid to argue about a punishment? [Each child spontaneously or in response to the question states that it does not do any good to argue.]

Manny: But I do argue about it sometimes.

Dr. A.:   Does it do you any good?

Manny: Not usually.

Dr. A.:   Not usually? You mean it sometimes does do some good? We have to do something about that right now! It should never do you any good! We have to do something about that right now. (*turning to Mr. I.*) Don't ever reduce a punishment when he argues with you about it. It's OK to get his opinion ahead of time. That's up to you. But once you have made your decision about the punishment, increase it rather than decrease it if he argues. For example, if he is restricted from his bicycle for one day and he argues, make it two days.

Mr. I.:   (*smiling*) In other words, negotiate in reverse? [Dr. A. nods, and Manny smiles.]

Why is Manny smiling? Is he masochistic? Does he have a secret trick up his sleeve? Is he paranoid? Is it a "scripty smile"? Although we cannot prove it, we have seen such a smile in similar situations with other children often enough that we believe it is a smile of relief. A child who has been in a position of questionable controls and limits often smiles when the parent is told in front of the child to crack down.

Dr. A.:   (*to Mr. I.*) Once you make the decision, it's not negotiable, and if he argues about it, it should be increased. Start low enough so that you can increase it if he tries to argue about it. [Here Dr. A. tries to program a more lenient initial punishment into the punitive Mr. I.'s response pattern under the guise of getting tough.] Manny, I know you're probably not very happy about what I'm saying, but this is the way it has to be. [Manny grins and continues to act friendly toward Dr. A.] Is there anyone else here who ever argues about a punishment? I can tell your parents the same thing if you want me to. [Group laughter.] Rick, how about you?

Rick: Well, usually not, but once in a while I argue about it.

Dr. A.:   (*turning to Rick's mother*) I'll tell you the same thing I told Mr. and Mrs. I.. If Rick argues about the punishment once you decide on it, increase it a little bit. It's okay to get his opinion about it before you make the decision or ask him what he thinks would be a good punishment or ask him to name the punishment, but once you make the final decision, no argument is allowed. Kurt, how about you?

Kurt: Well, once in a while I argue. (*looks at his mother sheepishly and snuggles into her arm*)

Dr. A.: (*looking at Kurt's mother*) You heard what I told the others. [She nods and smiles as Kurt smiles.]

Manny was given the strong message in a manner that was detoxified by having it addressed to him as part of a peer group. His somewhat hostile relationship with his father was possibly mellowed a bit by having the heavy message come from the psychiatrist rather than from his father and by taking external pressure off the father to negotiate while giving the father an incentive to start a bit lower on the penalty scale. The appeal to Mr. I. to modify his rigid sense of justice was done separately from the children so that he would not feel trapped or embarrassed in front of his son.

Defining a Good Punishment

Here is another excerpt from a parents' and children's discussion on punishment. Since many children and their parents do not have a clear understanding of the dynamics and purpose of punishment, the conversation focused on what are the most effective punishments and how children can prevent themselves from receiving a punishment or a worse punishment.

Dr. A.: Can any of you kids tell me what a good punishment is?

David: If you do something bad and you're not allowed to watch TV?

Dr. A.: Oh, you mean using TV as a punishment would be good? If you do something bad or don't do something you're supposed to do, then you're not allowed to watch something you would like to. Do you think that's a good punishment? Is it a good way to punish?

Kurt: You mean you couldn't watch your favorite program?

Dr. A.: Has that ever happened to you?

Kurt: On Sunday once.

Dr. A.:	Is that a good punishment? [The children look bewildered.] Is it a good way to punish? [They still seem unsure.] What is a good punishment?
Tom:	One that really hurts a lot. One that anybody would hate to have happen.
Dr. A.:	What if it was so bad that it got somebody discouraged and they gave up trying and did the bad thing again. Would that be a good punishment?
Paul:	No.
Dr. A.:	How else could we tell a good punishment? [No answer from the children.] How about the adults here? Who can say what a good punishment would be? [No answer from the parents.] Let's check with our high-priced help. How about you professionals?
Medical student:	You can tell by whether it is effective.
Dr. A.:	And what do you mean by effective?
Medical student:	Whether it keeps the kid from doing the same bad thing again.
Dr. A.:	Right! And that gives you kids some important information. Your parents are likely to decide that something is good punishment if it keeps you from doing the same bad thing again. Right? [Everyone nods.] And if they decide something is not a good punishment, what are they likely to do?
Paul and Kurt:	Give a worse punishment.
Dr. A.:	Right! So what's a good way to keep them from giving you a worse punishment?
Kurt:	Behave good after the first punishment.
Dr. A.:	Right! The smart thing for you to do is to prove to your parents that the easier punishment is a good one by showing that it works, that it keeps you from doing the bad thing again. Then you'll only have to have easy punishments.

Mrs. E.: One thing I don't understand is this: If television is a bad thing for them [Kurt is her son], does it make sense to have it be a punishment to take away from them?

Dr. A.: I see your point. If you decide that they should not see television anyhow, then that's not really a punishment.

Mrs. E.: Oh, I guess it could be that there are certain programs that you decide are OK for the kids to watch and that you would let them watch but you can take away those programs as a punishment.

Dr. A.: Right, even though the other programs, the bad ones, you would not let them watch regardless of whether they behave well or badly.

Mrs. E.: Okay, I understand now. I was a little confused about it at first, but it makes sense now.

Hurting with Love

In this third excerpt, Mr. Q. had been complaining that his son, Kevin, did not respond to any punishments, including corporal punishment, isolation, and taking away a favorite toy. Mr. Q. was convinced that he had exhausted all efforts and there was little that he could do. As the discussion continued, it became clear that Mr. Q's major problem was not one of finding a severe enough punishment for Kevin but in accepting his right as a parent to punish and set limits. Dr. A. did not yet know that as this vignette began:

Dr. A.: (*to Mr. Q.*) Kids like this have frustrated the most effective punishers, so don't feel like a failure because you're not able to get to him. One of the typical things reported is that hyperkinetic kids don't learn from punishments. You punish them and they go right back to it. This is a typical story. It seems that whatever it is in their brain, it is not connecting right; it has to do with the punishment center or with learning. They just don't seem to learn from punishment. It's often kind of a futile effort. Fortunately you can often get through to them by reinforcing them with rewards. What you do is reward the competing behavior. If they track mud in every day, you probably won't get very far if you punish. But if you start rewarding them for taking their shoes off and leaving them at the door, then they'll probably start leaving them there because rewards mean more than punishment.

Mr. Q.: Yeah, I'm constantly threatening him, "If you don't do such and such, you can't have _____." I'm just fed up.

Dr. E.: It makes a difference, too, on how you word what you're trying to convey. For example, you could say, "From now on you will need to earn your ice cream. As of now you no longer have the privilege of going to the refrigerator whenever you want. But you can do some things to earn the ice cream. Here are the things you can do . . ."

Mr. Q.: (*shaking his head no*) If he gets the ice cream, I'm not going to stop him. I just can't take it away from him.

Dr. E.: Well, it's really important for you to control the goodies.

Dr. A.: Can't you pull the ice cream from his hands? Do you feel like this would be denying him? In your house, you feel it is essential that everyone is entitled to ice cream?

Mr. Q.: Well, once he's got it.

Dr. A.: What about this? If he stole $10 and spent $1 of it, would you take the other $9 back?

Mr. Q.: Oh, yes, without question.

Dr. A.: Well, is it that you don't want the ice cream to go to waste? You could put it back in the refrigerator, couldn't you? Next time he's entitled, this is the one he gets.

Dr. E.: (*interrupting Dr. A. to Mr. Q.*) I think what Dr. A. is trying to say is that his rewards should be contingent on his behavior, so we don't allow freebies. I realize it's hard to crack down. Every parent likes to give their child things.

Mr. Q.: Well, you just want to give your kids more than you had as a child.

Dr. E.: That's beautiful on your part; however, you don't want to take it to the extreme. You shouldn't think you have to give him everything because you were deprived as a child. In some situations, he will deserve lots of goodies, and in some situations he won't.

Mr. Q.:   What if he hurts himself if I don't give it to him?

Dr. A.:   You're afraid that he's going to harm himself if you punish him? I think you'll do more harm in the long run if you let him get away with it for fear of him hurting himself than if you would refuse what he wants. Right now he throws himself on the floor but maybe in ten years he'll use a knife and OD on some pills. That's what happens. It escalates; the price keeps going up.

After the children returned from their separate group, the parents' conversation was adapted to the children:

Dr. A.:   OK, kids, now let's talk for a minute about something that the parents were worried about in the parents' group. I guess something that keeps coming up is how parents get kids to do things they ought to do or not do things they shouldn't do. I think you guys have been here long enough to figure this out. What are the two main ways? [No response from the children.] How about reward and punishment? You get a reward when you do the right things, and you get a punishment if you do wrong things.

Kurt: I don't get a reward when I clean my room.

Dr. A.:   Maybe your reward is having a clean room. Did you ever think that some rewards come so often that you don't think of them as rewards? I'd like to ask you guys something. I bet you'll be really surprised to find out what your parents talked about. What do you think? Would your parents rather reward or punish you?

Kurt: Reward!

Dr. A.:   Parents would rather reward you! Why?

Kurt: Because you clean your room.

Dr. A.:   That's right! If you clean your room, it makes them feel like rewarding you. Why would parents not want to punish you? Did you know that a lot of parents don't like to punish you? Why wouldn't they? It doesn't hurt them, does it?

Three children: Yes! [Note how a provocative question brought to the children's awareness a fact that is well known to adults but not ordinarily known to children: that it hurts parents to punish their children.]

Kurt: It hurts their hands.

Dr. A.:   OK. That could be. Are there any other ways it may hurt them?

Children: It could hurt their feelings.

Dr. A.:   Why would it hurt their feelings if they punish you? [No response.] No ideas?

Kurt: Because you're their son!

Dr. A.:   Right! Because you're their son. They don't like to see you hurt. You know it can be a problem for some parents. Maybe they want so much for you to have good things, they want to protect you. But maybe some parents let kids have too much or they don't punish them enough.

Tom: You mean spoil 'em?

Kurt: What would be bad about being spoiled?

Dr. A.:   You tell me. Would you like to be spoiled? [No one says yes.] None of you would like to be spoiled? Every once in a while you ask a kid and he says yes. They think that it would be great. So you kids think that it wouldn't be good for you to have everything? Why not?

Kevin: Kids would call you spoiled.

Dr. A.:   You mean other people wouldn't like you? [Kevin nods.] Also, if your parents spoil you, you would never learn how to save. You wouldn't learn good habits. How about this: you all agree that it's a good thing not to be spoiled and not have everything you want, but suppose there is something you want and mother and father say you can't have it?

Kurt: (*smiling*) Well, I guess that's the breaks.

Dr. A.:	That's the breaks? You would take that? You wouldn't get mad or yell? How about the rest of you kids? Kevin, how about you? What do you think about that?
Kevin:	If they said I couldn't have something, I'd get mad.
Dr. A.:	Do you think your parents would give it to you if you got mad?
Kevin:	You bet!
Dr. A.:	(*to Kevin*) Well, shame on them! What about the rest of you kids? Would your parents give it to you if you got mad?
Howie:	No.
Dr. A.:	Kevin, maybe we ought to ask your mother and father if they'd give it to you if you got mad. Let's check with them to make sure. [Dr. A. is trying to frame Kevin's parents into making a public commitment to stop reinforcing tantrums.]
Mrs. Q.:	No, I wouldn't give it to him.
Mr. Q.:	Well, that's why we're here—to find out what to do with him. [Mr. Q. sidesteps the frame, but Dr. A. does not give up.]
Dr. A.:	Since you brought him to find out what to do, I'll give you my opinion: I don't think you should give it to him if he acts that way.
Mr. E.:	This used to happen with Kurt, even in public, like in a restaurant. What we figured out is to leave the bad kid at home. No need to deprive the whole family of enjoying a good meal. I learned if I let him behave like that, I was bound to resent him. [Mr. E. had been attending for over six months and had become a cotherapist.]
Dr. A.:	That's a good example of the need for parents to insist on some reasonable rights. If you don't, you'll resent the child for violating your rights, and it's hard to be a good parent

while resenting. So to be a good parent, you have to insist that your child respect your rights.

Mr. Q. felt that if he were to punish Kevin, he would be depriving him of the things he was deprived of as a child. He apparently needed external support to feel justification in punishing Kevin. Dr. A. and Dr. E. attempted to shoulder the psychological burden of being the heavy by instructing Mr. Q. in front of his son and the rest of the group, but Mr. Q. was not receptive. Finally, with the help of Mr. E., Dr. A. tried to rechannel his guilt in the service of being firm, setting limits, and realizing his parental duty.

22
Lying

Behavior-disordered children are often considered bad by parents, teachers, and neighbors. Some parents tend to define the problem as one of morality. One of the contributing factors is that such children often lag behind age-mates in their progression of moral development, as well as other areas of development. It is important to help the parents see that this moral immaturity is as much a handicap as the child's cognitive, emotional, behavioral, physical, and sometimes anatomical immaturity. The concept of stage development is often useful in explaining the child's lag. This has the advantage of offering hope for the child to achieve a more mature and moral level of functioning in the future.

Parents have three common complaints: (1) lying, which may result from delay in concrete operational thinking; (2) unaltruistic motivation (selfishness), normal for younger children; and (3) stealing, often as an attempt to maintain some control over the environment and obtain rewards from a world from which the child has not been able to obtain reinforcements in honest ways with the same ease as normal children. The following example illustrates how these problems can be addressed in multifamily group.

Three parents brought up the topic of lying. Tony's mother complained that Tony lied all the time even when it was not necessary. Kurt and Tom's father reported defensive lying as a problem, though he did not use those words. He described each lying to deny what he had done after the other one reported him. The brothers would often also get into arguments as to who had done something wrong, each denying it ("lying about it"). Three-and-one-half-year-old Kevin's mother reported that he did a lot of lying in the sense of making up stories about things that happened to get attention and increase his importance. Dr. A. responded to the parents' concerns about lying with the following minilecture, a bit longer than most:

Dr. A.:   Have we talked recently about different kinds of lying and reasons for them? [All the parents look puzzled, and a few shake their heads no.] The reasons for lying vary somewhat and partly depend on the age of the child. For example, below the age of six, a child is not able to appreciate another point of view; he has ego-centric thinking, and therefore he is not able to think about the possibility of deceiving someone else. If he tells something that is not so, it's not with the intention to deceive and is therefore not a lie in the moral sense. It's really more of a wish expression or a fantasy expression. If you see him break something and ask, "Did you break that?" and he says "no," what he really means is, "I wish I hadn't broken it," or possibly he uses the denial as a sort of magic incantation that may ward off punishment, especially if he has found on a a few occasions in the past that denial would get him out of a punishment. But a preschool child doesn't really expect that he can prevent you from knowing what he knows merely by denying it. He thinks you already know. The solution to this kind of lying, of course, is not to give him the opportunity. Don't ask him if you know for sure he did something. Tell him, "You broke that, and you will therefore have to give up this" or whatever action you feel you should take.

Children above the age of six gradually develop the ability to understand another person's point of view and to appreciate the fact that they might be able to deceive you since you don't know the same things they do, and they don't know the same things you do. The most common form of lying in the school age group is defensive lying: lying to get out of the consequence of something, usually to get out of a punishment or to get out of an embarrassing situation. The answer to this is to make sure there is not a greater penalty for telling the truth than there is for lying. This can get a little bit tricky, because if a child can avoid a bad consequence one time out of ten by lying and doesn't get any worse punishment if he lies than if he tells the truth, he gets intermittently reinforced for lying. This is only common sense. After all, if you have a chance for a payoff one time and it doesn't cost you anything to keep trying, naturally you will keep trying. Defensive lying in this kind of a situation is merely a sign of intelligence.

In order to punish more severely for lying about something, you first have to make sure the youngster really is lying. Therefore you should not ask except in situations where you already know for sure or have some other way of checking on it. In doubtful situations it may be better not to ask, because if the youngster denies, then you're trapped between two bad choices: either punishing for the lie as well as the act and possibly erroneously in case the child did not do it, or on the other hand accepting the denial and thereby reinforcing the lie.

Another form of lying is ego building. This isn't too far different than fish stories and involves bragging in an exaggerated way that departs from the truth. This is not unusual for very young children and in many cases can merely be ignored. If it gets too far out of hand, it can be dealt with through such a statement as, "It would be nice if you really could do that kind of thing," or, "It's nice to imagine that you can do things like that," or, "It's fun to imagine that you can do things like that, isn't it?" which indicates the child's degree of exaggeration is not acceptable, but his desire to bolster his self-esteem or win attention and admiration is understandable.

Another form of lying is sabotaging or malicious, in which one lies to get a rival in trouble. This type of lying will extinguish itself if it is not reinforced by action against the rival whom the youngster is attempting to get in trouble. If it is too excessive or frequent to be ignored, then it should be firmly limited and even punished if necessary. One good way to do this is to couple siblings in a buddy system where if one is punished, the other one is also punished, which takes away the incentives for tattling.

After the children returned from their separate group, the topic was adapted as follows:

Dr. A.:   All right, we've talked about what you kids did in your separate group; now let's talk about something the parents talked about in their group. One of the things that I think you kids will be interested in is lying. What do you think about lying? Is it good or bad, or does it make any difference? [Three children say "bad," and the other three nod their heads in agreement.] What is so bad about it? What makes lying bad? [Two children put up their hands.] Bill?

Bill: Because you can get in bigger trouble if you lie.

Dr. A.:   That's right. You can get in bigger trouble for lying than if you didn't lie. Do the rest of you agree with that? [Other children nod or say yes.] In fact, that's what happened with President Nixon, why he almost went to jail. It was mostly for lying, for trying to cover up what his men did. He had to stop being president and almost went to jail because of lying, and if he had told the truth in the first place, he would probably have been able to keep on being president to the end of his term. So lying can get you in bigger trouble. But is that the only thing wrong with lying? Is there anything else bad about it? Kurt?

Kurt: You might feel bad about it inside.

Dr. A.: Right! After you tell a lie or do anything else bad, you feel bad in-side about it. How many people here can remember ever feeling bad about something that you did that you shouldn't have? [Five of the children and three or four adults raise their hands. The sixth child looks hesitant and puzzled, with his hand in an am-biguous position. Dr. A. takes the opportunity to nudge this child's ambivalence in the right direction.] It's normal to feel bad after you do something wrong. That's what helps us remember to keep from making the same mistake again the next time. Of course, it's not just enough to feel bad about it. We also have to make a plan about how we're going to do the right thing the next time. But is there any other bad thing about lying?

Tony: If you lie, nobody will like you, and you won't have any friends. [Two other children nod, and one says, "oh yeah."]

Dr. A.: Is it important to have friends? Do you want to have friends? [All children nod or say yes.] And would lying make people want to stop being your friend? [All the children nod or say yes.] Is there anything else bad about lying? [Four children fall silent and look pensive; Tony begins fidgeting; three-and-a-half-year-old Kevin begins whispering in his mother's ear. Dr. A. realizes the need to engage more right-brain function to hold their attention.] Did you ever hear the story about the boy who cried "wolf?" [All children's interest perks up.]

Kurt: You told that story a long time ago, when I first came here.

Dr. A.: It looks like the other kids haven't heard it, though, so could you tell it for them?

Kurt: You're the one who told it in the first place. (*seems reluctant and unsure*) [Kurt, though obviously remembering the story and able to tell it, seems hindered by a mild degree of stage fright. To relieve the tension, Dr. A. switches to a humorous reassurance that Kurt can tell the story as well as he.]

Dr. A.: But would you tell it this time? I'm getting old—I'm over eigh-teen—and my memory is getting bad. I'm not sure I can remember it. [Laughter from the whole group.]

Kurt: (*immensely enjoying the joke, confers briefly with his father, then with a sly grin says*) That was a fib!

Dr. A.:   That's right, Kurt! It was a fib in a way because my memory is not that bad. It is true that I am getting older [more laughter], but my memory isn't that bad yet. But I wanted you to tell the story for the other kids, so I made kind of a joke out of it.

Kurt: That was just a little white lie.

Dr. A.:   There's a difference between a joking fib and serious lie. How can you tell which it is?

Kurt: You could tell by the smile on the person's face when they tell a joking fib.

Dr. A.:   Good. That's one way. Does anybody else have any ideas about the difference?

Bill: If everybody laughs, you know it's not really a lie; it's just a joke.

Dr. A.:   That's right. Every joke is a lie in a way, because it's really a story that's just made up, not something that really happened. For example, you might start out, "There were these two guys named Tweedle Dee and Tweedle Dum that were walking over a bridge." Now there really weren't any guys named Tweedledee and Tweedledum, but everybody understands that you are just making that up to tell the joke, and that's not really a lie. What is the difference between that and the lie? [The children look perplexed and pensive. One begins to fidget again. Dr. A. decides to supply the answer while they are still receptive.] The difference is that in a serious lie, you are trying to fool the other person; you are trying to make the other person believe something that's not true. But in a joking fib, you are not really trying to make the other person believe something that's not true; you want him to understand that you are just making it up for a joke. Do you all understand that difference? [They all nod, four of them with a look of understanding.]

How should Dr. A. proceed now? Ordinarily it would have been advisable to ask one of the children to repeat the explanation to make sure that they understood; however, Dr. A. was concerned that the children had twice indicated their waning of interest and felt it best to proceed with the story.

Dr. A.: OK, Kurt, are you ready to tell the story now about the boy who cried "wolf?"

Kurt: (*with a bit more assurance and in a more relaxed manner than when he had first been asked to tell it*) I'll tell the story, and you tell the moral.

Dr. A.: OK.

Kurt: Well, there was this boy who was supposed to watch the sheep and he got bored and cried "wolf." Well, you see, he was supposed to call "wolf" whenever a wolf came, and the townspeople would come out with guns to kill the wolf. But he would call "wolf" when there really was not a wolf, and everybody came out running and were mad at him when they found out there really was no wolf. Then he did it a second time because he liked the excitement, and then the third time they said they wouldn't come anymore. And then finally when the wolf really did come and he cried "wolf," nobody would come out because they didn't believe him, and the wolf ate up all the sheep.

Dr. A.: And that's one of the most important reasons why lying is bad: if you lie sometimes, then when you need to have people believe you when you're telling the truth, they might not believe you.

Tony: (*to Dr. A.*) Now you tell the moral.

Bill: He did!

Tony: Oh, yes . . .

Dr. A.: I just did: if you want people to believe you when you need to have them believe you, you need to tell the truth at other times too.

Dr. A. took the opportunity to restate the moral in the converse form so that the children would have two different chances to understand it.

23
Stealing

L ying and stealing seem to be the two "moral" problems most destructive of parent-child trust. Lying was treated in the previous chapter; stealing is considered here. As with other morally immature behavior, there are many possible underlying reasons. When families become aware of the reasons for such unacceptable behavior, often they are able to devise means of dealing with it. The following transcript shows one way to cultivate awareness by both parents and children. This interaction occurred in the last segment following a parents' group in which the topic had been stealing by children.

Dr. A.:   Now that you kids have reported on what happened in your group, I'd like to report on something from parents' group: stealing. What is stealing? [Several hands go up.] Marge?

Marge: Taking something that doesn't belong to you.

Dr. A.:   Right. Why would somebody do that?

Frank: They don't have something.

Frank's mother: Talk louder, Frank. No one can hear you.

Dr. A.:   I understood what he meant. He said they want something they don't have.

Paul: Maybe they ain't sure other kids believe him.

Paul's mother: (*correcting Paul's grammar*) Maybe they *aren't* sure other kids believe *them*.

Dr. A.:   I don't think the grammar is important here. The important thing is that they can say what they're thinking. [Twice now Dr. A. has had to intervene to protect a child's spontaneity from a parent's good-intentioned but ill-timed correction. Finally the parents take the cue and enjoy the following interaction.] Paul said they sometimes take things to prove to other kids that they can do it. Isn't that what you said?

Paul: Because somebody called him a name like *chicken.*

Sam: They have a temptation.

Dr. A.:   Oh, somebody or something tempts them to do it. The kid acts kind of like the devil encourages him to do something wrong. Those sound like a lot of good ideas. Maybe some of the other kids have ideas about it, too. [Four of the eight children present have contributed thus far. Dr. A. has just invited the others to follow the lead; however, they merely look pensive and hesitant. He gives them time to formulate ideas by using the time to summarize and credit the ideas so far offered. This process might also provoke more tangential ideas, consolidate the insights established, and reinforce through attention and approval those who have already spoken.] I think there are lots of different reasons people do things. One person might steal for one reason and another for another reason. Frank gave one reason: that maybe they want something, have a desire for it. Paul said that maybe they're challenged or dared to do it. Somebody says, "I bet you're chicken to steal that," or "I bet you can't do it," so they take the dare and go ahead and do it. Another reason was given by Sam: maybe they want something they don't have, and the only way they can think of to get it is to steal it. OK. What are some other reasons? Do any of you other kids have ideas? [Children still look hesitant.] The parents can contribute, too, if they want to. Big people are allowed to chime in on this.

Marge's mother: Instead of stealing, you could ask for it.

Dr. A.:   That's very good, because maybe one reason some kids steal is that they don't think their mother or father would get something for them if they would ask.

Mike:	What if they say "no"?

Dr. A.:	Could you take a "no" if you were told "no"? Would you be able to give up on something? [Mike nods.] How about the rest of the kids? If your mother would tell you "no" on something you want? Maybe they can't afford it. Maybe you want a new bicycle and they can't afford to get it. Would you be able to take the "no"? [Most children nod, but George shakes his head.] You wouldn't, George? What would you do about it?

George:	(*mischievously*) I'd scream and yell and stomp.

How could Dr. A. respond to George? One way could be to pick up on George's attempted humor and carry it to absurdity in order to discredit screaming and stomping as a serious option: "Oh, you'd entertain your mother; you'd dance and sing like a rock star to earn what you want. [Turning to George's mother] Is he good enough at screaming and stomping to get what he wants?" His mother would undoubtedly laugh and indicate that she would not give in to the tantrum. If she wavers, she should be told firmly in front of the group never to give in. What Dr. A. actually did was to ignore the mischievousness and reframe George's statement as an admission of a problem—failure of self-control—to be empathized with:

Dr. A.:	You couldn't take it. You'd get mad. You know, one of the hard things in growing up is learning how to take "no" for an answer, because it is natural to get mad. [Here Dr. A. helps George feel accepted for being honest about his behavior. He interprets George's admission as a growing pain rather than a moral failing. Then he goes on to plant the idea of how troublesome the immature behavior is and how grown-up the desired adaptive behavior would be.] That's the natural thing for anybody who can't have what you want; you get mad. Or maybe you decide you are going to steal it and then get in trouble for that. But learning how to give up on something you can't get is one of the things in growing up. [Vince's hand up.] OK, what is it Vince?

Vince:	I aggravate Mom if she doesn't give it to me.

Dr. A.:	Can you get your mother to get you things by aggravating her? [Vince shakes head no.] OK, good for her. (*turning to*

other children) Vince said "no," and I said good for his mother, because they shouldn't get things for you for aggravating and annoying them because what would that do? If you could get what you wanted by aggravating and annoying, what would that do? [Frank's hand goes up first.]

Frank: You'd get in the habit.

Dr. A.:   That's right. You'd get in the habit of doing that. They would be teaching you to aggravate and annoy, and who wants to be an aggravating and annoying person when they grow up? [Mike, accompanied by his aunt because his mother could not get off work, raises his hand.]

Mike: My mother gives me something if I pester her long enough.

Dr. A.:   Oh, she does give it to you? Shame on her! Listen, would you give her a message from me that she shouldn't do that? (*looking around room*) If there are any mothers or fathers here who give kids what they want just because they get annoying, I'm telling you right now: don't do it, because you are teaching kids to be aggravating and annoying, and that's bad for the kids. (*turning back to Mike*) I'm going to ask your aunt also to give your mother the message. Maybe if both of you tell her, she'll listen to it. OK, Mike? [Mike grins.] Anybody have any other ideas why somebody would steal? Marge has her hand up and then Mrs. J.

Marge: Maybe they think it's theirs.

Dr. A.:   Oh, they might think it's theirs when they take it, but it really belongs to somebody else. Is that stealing, if you think it's yours? If you see something and you think it's yours but it really belongs to somebody else because it looks alike, and you take it, is that stealing? [Two hands go up, with head shaking.] Matt says no. Vince says no. What do you say?

Marge: Yeah, because you didn't ask them if it was theirs or not.

Dr. A.:   Oh, you should ask about it to check. What if you're sure of it, and it doesn't even occur to you that there is any chance it belongs to someone else?

Matt: You could save trouble by checking.

Dr. A.:   Matt has an idea: he's saying that even though that is not stealing and you're not a bad person for doing that, still you could prevent problems by checking. If you always check and make sure that it is yours, then you won't get in trouble, and you won't have to take it back to the person. That's a good thought, Matt. [Frank's hand up.] Frank?

Frank: A kid at school keeps taking my pencil, and he won't give it back. I show him where I put my name on it, but he won't give it back. I tell Mr. J., the teacher, but he won't do anything.

Dr. A.:   Did you tell your teacher that it had your name on it? [Frank nods.] And the teacher could see the name on it, and the teacher didn't make him give it back to you? [This may seem like a tangent, but watch where it leads. Dr. A. did not know when he started exploring Frank's complaint where it would lead but was confident that taking a sincere interest in a child's problem would be productive.]

Frank: He wouldn't admit it.

Dr. A.:   Who, the teacher?

Frank: No, my friend.

Dr. A.:   (*with amazement*) You mean it was a friend that stole your pencil? [Frank nods.] And he's still your friend?

Frank: Not any more.

Dr. A.:   Well, I guess not! That's one of the bad things about stealing. If you steal from a friend, you can lose a friend. I'm thinking of one other possible reason why somebody might steal, and that is that maybe they don't feel very sure that they'll have enough to live on.

Vince: If your electricity is turned off, maybe you need the money to pay the electric bill, so you can have electricity.

Dr. A.:   Sometimes people will steal because they are going to starve to death. If they can't steal what they need, they'll steal the money to go buy what they need. But sometimes

	people will steal when they think they need things, but they really don't need them. They feel so unsure inside themselves, they think the only way they can have anything for sure for themselves is by stealing. I think a lot of kids steal for that reason.
Marge's mother:	Maybe some kids steal because they think that's the only thing they do well.
Dr. A.:	That's another idea. [Vince's hand up.] Vince, do you have another one?
Vince:	They think it's funny, like taking somebody's hat.
Dr. A.:	You mean a joke or a prank. They call that a practical joke sometimes, but they're not really funny. They're kind of mean.
Frank:	You can take things back before you get caught.
Dr. A.:	That's right. Maybe somebody has stolen something, and you're sorry you stole it. Frank is saying then that the best thing to do is take it back because you can get out of trouble if you take it back. They won't blame you for it then. They'll usually forgive you, like in the store: if you pick up something in a store, usually if you take it back right away, they won't call the police or anything like that. That's a good idea, Frank. I'm really glad you brought that up. (*looking around the room approvingly and speaking to the adults*) The kids really have some good ideas. All of them contributed to the discussion.

Note that Dr. A. ended the discussion with reinforcement for the children's participation, which not only increases the frequency of future participation but also fortifies them for the feedback (positive and negative) immediately following.

Provocative Therapy

Children are naturals for a provocative therapy approach once they have taken a reasonable stand on some issue. As adapted to children, it combines elements of provocation, straw man technique, Socratic questioning, reverse consultation role playing, and devil's advocacy. The group leader takes the "wrong" side of a moral or judgment issue and allows the children to persuade him or her to switch over to the right side. This is illustrated in the following transcript vignette. All of the children's parents had stated in parents' group that each of them had lied or stolen or both.

Dr. A.: Now that you kids have told us about what you did in your group we need to tell you about something the parents were talking about in their group. They were talking about lying and stealing. Who can tell what lying is? [Two hands go up.] Tony?

Tony: Saying something that's not so.

Dr. A.: Right. And who can tell me what stealing is? [Jane's hand goes up.] Jane?

Jane: Taking something that does not belong to you.

Dr. A.: That's right. OK. Why do people do it? [Two hands go up.] Joe?

Joe: Because they want something and don't have the money to buy it.

Dr. A.: OK. That's one reason. Anything else?

Pat: Maybe somebody else stole something from them and they're trying to get even.

Tony: They shouldn't do it because it's wrong.

Dr. A.: Do all you kids agree with Tony? [All children nod in agreement.] You all agree you shouldn't lie or steal? [All nod again.] There must be some reason that kids do it because they're not dumb; they must get something good out of it. What can a person get out of it? What can a person get out of lying or stealing?

Jane: They can get grounded. [Laughter from whole group.]

Dr. A.: You mean they get in trouble?

Joe: Yes.

Dr. A.: But there must be something good about it or kids would never do it. It sounds to me like lying could be a good way of getting out of trouble if you did something wrong.

Jane: (*Warming to the argument*) But if you tell one lie, you have to tell another lie to cover that one up and then another lie, and pretty soon you get all mixed up.

Dr. A.: You mean you get caught in your own lies? [Several children nod] But what if you're real smart about it—maybe if you think out real carefully how to tell a good lie—then you wouldn't get caught in it. [The children look a little pensive for a few seconds and then two hands are raised.] Pat?

Pat: Somebody would find out after awhile and then people would not believe you anymore.

Dr. A.: Oh. Well, OK. I guess maybe lying is not a very good idea at that. I guess the people who tell lies just haven't figured out what's good for themselves. But what about stealing? Surely stealing could be a good way of getting what you want.

Several
kids: (*in unison*) No!

Dr. A.: Why not? If there's something you want, why not just take it?

Jane: When you get caught you'll just have to give it back or pay back and then maybe your mother or father will take something away from you to teach you a lesson, so you have less than what you started with.

Dr. A.: But at least you got to have it for a little while.

Pat: It's not worth it if you get punished. Besides, if you steal from a friend, they'll get mad at you.

Dr. A.: Why should they get mad at you?

Pat: Because you took something that belonged to them and then they don't have it anymore.

Tony: If there's something you want and don't have the money, you should ask your mother to get it for you or give you the money for it.

Dr. A.: But, what if she won't give it to you?

Tony: Then you'll have to wait until you get your allowance.

Dr. A.:   But suppose it's a long time 'til your allowance.

Tony: It might not be so long. If you get your allowance on Friday and it's Thursday, you would only have to wait a day.

Dr. A.:   But suppose it's Saturday and you get your allowance on Friday. Then you would have to wait a whole week.

Pat: Then you would have to suffer.

Dr. A.:   But who wants to suffer?

Jane: You would suffer more if you steal something and get caught.

Dr. A.:   Oh, well, I guess you kids have talked me out of it. I'm just going to have to mend my ways and not steal anymore. [Laughter from the whole group.]

The following points need to be noted about this technique.

1. The leader needs to indicate nonverbally that this is just "pretend" or teasing or joking and that the leader does not really believe in the position taken for the sake of argument.
2. It is important to bring up the "devil's arguments" that might appeal to a child in temptation, such as being able to have the use of the stolen object for immediate gratification.
3. Above all, it is important to let the children win the argument and to concede the argument explicitly so that they can identify with the right prevailing.
4. It is helpful to explore whether the child can use concrete operational thinking to appreciate the point of view of the victim, because this can give the child a more mature basis for the desired moral position. However, this is not necessary for the straw man indoctrination. In fact, many of the cogent arguments used above by the children depended on only an instrumental level of understanding, within the reach of preoperational thinking.

24
The Name and Blame Game with Chemical Consequences

Once children are diagnostically labeled, there is a tendency to blame everything that goes wrong on the disorder. A certain amount of this is desirable; insofar as parents and teachers need to assess any blame, it is better for them to blame the disorder than the child or each other. Often we see overkill, however. A parent may excuse a child from all responsibility for actions because he or she is "hyperkinetic" or "epileptic" or otherwise handicapped. A corollary is that some parents do not consider the problem adequately treated until the child has reached a standard of perfection that would be impossible even for normal, nonhandicapped children. This is one of the reasons that we repeatedly stress improvement rather than perfection as the standard of success in group.

Some people blame the child for being hyperkinetic, and some people excuse the child for being hyperkinetic.

Mrs. V.: I'm not sure I understand what this label is all about. Aren't there things that children do that are just natural for all children? Shouldn't they be punished for some things? We can't always blame what a child does on hyperactivity, can we?

Dr. A.: That's a good point, but it's not clear to me whether your question regards punishment. Do you think that whether his [Paul's] behavior is due to hyperactivity determines whether you should punish him?

Mrs. V.: I'm not sure. If other boys do those things, aren't they hyperactive?

Mrs. E.: You get tired of deciding if it's hyperactive behavior or not!

Mrs. T.: I used to have grand mal seizures. My parents got caught up in me being sick and treated me as a "sicky" all through my life. I wasn't treated as normal, so I want to treat David as normal.

Dr. E.:   One of the problems we run into is thinking in terms of good or bad, all or none. In answer to your questions, any child will fail to complete his homework or get wound up at times. One of the factors in deciding whether your child's behavior is hyperactive is how often it happens.

Dr. A.:   The problem is when we get hung up on normal and abnormal. We should be concentrating on what we can do to help the child improve his behavior. If a child cannot take responsibility, then a mother should temporarily take it in terms of setting limits. You're taking responsibility for him until he develops it himself. Whether he's diagnosed as hyperactive doesn't really matter.

Dr. E.:   Labels can be self-perpetuating, like a bureaucracy. Once a kid gets a label, regardless of the type of label, there is a tendency to see everything he does in light of that behavior.

Dr. A.:   We must remember, too, that each hyperactive child is different; however, techniques that have been successful in managing behavior for hyperactive children are the same as those with normal children.

The labeling and blaming issue naturally leads into the medication issue for several reasons: some people assume that if a diagnosis is made, there should be some medicine prescribed; some people see medication as a kind of punishment or discipline; and some people see medication as a kind of chemical morality or magic that will eliminate blame and perfect the child. It is not surprising that a question about medication immediately followed in this same session.

Mrs. T.:   How do you feel about medication?

Dr. A.:   If a child is in danger of flunking out of school because of high distractibility, attention deficit, or overactive impulsiveness, then it may be necessary and beneficial. But even some kids with those problems in school can be helped without medication. For example, one of the kids with a memory and attention problem has improved in school after memory practice here in the group. Occasionally, we give medicine to kids that are hard to like so that they can behave in a way that allows them to experience their parents' love. Parents' love is an essential nutrient for growing children.

Mrs. T.: I don't want to put my son on medication just because I can't deal with him.

Mrs. E.: But you're the one who has to deal with him. I didn't want to put Kurt on medication, but . . .

Mrs. T.: Maybe I see him differently than others, though. Maybe it's just me, and I shouldn't medicate him.

Dr. A.: That's a good point: you shouldn't just medicate the child without making any changes in your handling of him. But don't overdo your responsibility in the relationship with him. It reminds me of what some people have said about school. If the child isn't adjusting in school, then the school should make the adjustments. That's not exactly how it works. Everyone may have to make adjustments: school, parents, and child, maybe even other family members.

Mrs. T.: I'm just afraid of medication, and I want to try other routes first.

Mrs. E.: But you have to get through now.

Here is a good illustration of a parent's having the freedom to tell another parent things that would be difficult for a professional, who might seem to have an axe to grind. Because of her own childhood role as a medicated epileptic, Mrs. T. was conflicted about medication and needed some assurance that it would be all right to give her son medicine if necessary. Mrs. E. provides enough medication advocacy that the leader was relieved of that responsibility, which would have been awkward and less effective. He had the luxury of the following approach:

Dr. A.: Mrs. T. has a good point. Any medicine, even aspirin, carries some risk and should only be used for good reason. Of course, there is also a risk in not using it if it's needed, but we generally favor her idea of trying other things first. That's why I rarely prescribe medicine at the first visit. It often turns out to be unnecessary. In fact, there may be some children who would not even be helped by medicine but get better with the other things we do here. We need to balance the odds—the risks and possible benefits—and decide what order to try things in. Of course, any treatment that we might recommend for a child, including medication, the parent has a veto over.

After the children returned, the excuse topic was reintroduced.

Dr. A.: One of the things we talked about in the parents' group was parents making excuses for you because you're hyper and then parents don't expect things from you. Does that ever happen—that you and your parents make excuses for you? Kurt, can you tell us when you have used it as an excuse?

Kurt: (*shakes his head no and indignantly decides he does not wish to respond*)

Paul: Sometimes I tell my sister I'm hyper; then I smile.

Dr. A.: Isn't that teasing? [Paul nods affirmatively.] Is it true that children with hyperkinesis do things impulsively without thinking?

Kurt: Yes.

Paul: If they drink pop, they'll be hyper.

Dr. A.: Are you saying, then, it's an excuse for your behavior? When you don't behave or you get in trouble, do you use it as an excuse to get out of it?

Paul: It's an excuse.

Dr. A.: So what does that mean you have to do?

Paul: Maybe get hyper pills?

Dr. A.: There are other ways to get around this besides using pills. Maybe you have to try harder to work on your behavior—devise a plan to make changes and practice doing it. Some guys have trouble paying attention to things, remembering things, or even controlling their temper. They think it won't ever get better, so they give up without even trying. Well, the same way you can learn to run or swim, you can learn to control your temper or improve your attention or memory.

Dr. E. shifts some of the focus back to the parents in an effort to help the parents and children feel together in the problem and to help redefine the parent's role as a supportive assistant and coach through adversity. Mrs. J. responds by some genuine sharing, with which Dr. A. is then able to empathize:

Dr. E.: Part of the job of a parent, perhaps, is to keep the child from giving up.

Mrs. J.: The hardest thing for us was trying to keep from being resentful.

Dr. A.: I guess the whole situation seems unfair. It's no one's fault, but at times it does feel unfair. To keep from taking resentment out on each other is important.

In contrast to Mrs. T.'s skepticism, some parents are so sold on the benefits of medication that they tend to blame any problem the child has onto a medication deficiency of some kind: a skipped dose, need for an increased dosage, need for a change of medicine, or other implication that more medicine would be the answer. This assumption is based partly on the belief that anything the child does wrong is a product of the disorder. The following vignette illustrates a deterioration in child behavior that is actually a normal response to stress but was mistakenly interpreted by his mother as a flare-up of attention deficit disorder requiring an increase in medication. This session occurred the first week of January.

Mrs. H.: Zeke has been terrible the past week. I would like somebody to take a look at his medication after the group. He has gotten along very well the past five months since starting the medicine, but the past three weeks he has been terrible, and I think it might be wearing off. Maybe he needs a higher dose.

Dr. A.: Someone can meet with you afterwards to discuss that, but is it possible that something else has influenced his behavior recently?

Mrs. H.: I don't think so.

Dr. A.: Has anybody died, been sick, moved? Any other changes in his routine? Change of school or anything else? And, of course, the Christmas holidays affect some children.

Mrs. H.: Well, his grandfather died, but that was in November, and he should be over that by now.

Mrs. I.: Kids take a long time to get over things like that. Was he very attached to his grandfather?

Mrs. H.: Yes; since we moved back to town, he has spent a lot of time with him. And of course I was sort of at a loss for a while when he died. One other thing: do you think it could have anything to do with his father being away at school in Colorado for two weeks? This is the second week that he has been gone.

Mrs. Y.: It sounds like he has had a lot of things happening to him in the past month or so that could be upsetting him: his grandfather died, there was the excitement of Christmas, and now his father being away for a while.

Dr. A.: Have you talked with him about these things?

Mrs. H.: No, I guess I didn't think about this, but I can see how maybe these other things have been upsetting him more than usual.

Later in the same group, when it was time for choosing assignments for the coming week, Zeke was not sure what to take. At the suggestion of Mr. V. (one of the other parents) he agreed to take as his project to help clean up the house in preparation for his father's return in four days. He would help make a list of the work that needed to be done, choose one or two tasks to do himself, assign one or two tasks to his older brother, and ask his mother to take care of the rest. His oppositional behavior mellowed considerably at that point. In subsequent weeks Mrs. H. reported improvement in Zeke's behavior, without increased dosage.

25
Apologies

pologies are difficult for anyone, and especially for children. Consequently, parents often face situations where it is obvious that children should apologize, but they do not. There are two schools of thought about coercing apologies. One is that a forced apology is not sincere, is therefore meaningless, and is a violation of the child's integrity. The other school of thought is that going through the motions of apologizing has some value, at least in the sense of desensitizing the child to this uncomfortable chore. In addition, cognitive dissonance may produce some genuine contrition after the fact. Finally, there may be some aversive value to the embarrassment of a forced apology that may be not only more effective but more appropriate than some unrelated punishment. On balance, our sympathies drift in the direction of allowing forced apologies as long as one realizes that it is an imperfect undertaking.

Another area of possible disagreement about managing children's apologies is how much responsibility the parents should take. Should they apologize for their son or daughter? Should they even perhaps shoulder some of the child's guilt, as Bill's mother seems to want to do in the following transcript? Some subtle ramifications of this issue that are not immediately apparent are explored in the transcript. During this exploration, Dr. A. became aware of some considerations that changed his mind.

This transcript is from the last parent-child segment of a group. Eight children from seven families were present. One of the interesting aspects of this group was the free-flowing participation of both children and parents. Sometimes this segment of the group is merely a Socratic discussion between the group leader and various children. Rarely is it dominated by parents. Such unbalanced discussions have value, but when appropriate, it is desirable to involve both generations for a true multifamily group.

Dr. A.: Let's switch over now to what we talked about in the parents' group. One of the things that you kids might find very interesting is the idea of parents apologizing for their kids' behavior. I'd like to hear what the kids think about that. If you do something wrong like hurt somebody else, cause a fuss, make a scene in public, or do something embarrassing and cause somebody else some trouble, do you think your parents should apologize for you? [Scott shakes his head no.] You don't think so, Scott?

Scott: Yeah.

Dr. A.: Oh, you think they should? [Tricia's hand up.] Tricia, what do you think?

Tricia: The one who does it should apologize.

Dr. A.: The one who does it should apologize? The parents shouldn't apologize?

Tricia: Yeah. The parents shouldn't be the ones. The kid shouldn't get away with it. [Bill's hand up.]

Dr. A.: Bill?

Bill R.: I should apologize and not my mother.

Mrs. R.: But I also want to apologize. I feel like my family has hurt somebody by the public fuss, and I should apologize.

Dr. A.: (*to Bill*) So it sounds like she's not wanting you to take this job away from her. She's wanting to apologize, too. What do you think about that?

Bill: I don't know.

Dr. A.: Maybe some of the other kids could answer. Scott, you thought the parents should apologize. Do you think the kids should apologize also? [Scott nods.] What if a kid apologizes first? Does a parent then have to? [Scott shakes head no.] Oh, then you think it's not necessary for the parent to apologize. [Barbara's hand up.] OK, Barbara, what do you think?

Barbara: I don't think they should apologize.

Dr. A.: You think the kid should and not the parent? [Barbara nods; Jeff's hand up.] Jeff, what do you think?

Jeff: The kid.

Dr. A.: You think the kid should apologize and not the parent. [Jeff nods.] Why not the parent? Some of the kids say the parents should not apologize. [Tim's hand up.] What do you think, Tim?

Tim: It's not the parent's fault if a kid does something wrong. The kid should apologize.

Mrs. R.: I've been in the situation where you can see something happen before the child sees it was wrong. You as the parent can point it out to the child and let him know.

Dr. A.: You think the child has the responsibility, but the parent should still apologize?

Mrs. R.: I guess so.

Dr. A.: Let's find out from some of the other kids who have not answered. Todd, what about you?

Todd: The kids.

Dr. A.: OK. How about you, Kim?

Kim: Both.

Dr. A.: Oh, you think the kid should apologize and so should the parent. It looks like we kind of have a split in opinion. [Bill's hand up.] Bill, did you want to say something?

Bill: They both should.

Dr. A.: You've kind of changed your mind. At first you said just the kids should apologize and not the parents. Do you think you are influenced by what your mother says? Because maybe she would want to apologize for you?

Mrs. R.: I was saying that if he apologized on his own, OK, but if, say, he smashed a window and somebody tells me, then I think I should say, "I'm very sorry that happened, and I'm sure Bill is sorry. I'll see that something is done about it."

Dr. A.:   Can you really say that somebody else is sorry? [Bill's mother looks nonplussed. Dr. A. feels he has accomplished his purpose and shifts the focus to let her save face.] Let me ask some other questions: What if a kid will not apologize? Some of you think that the kid should apologize, but what if he won't?

Bill: He should do it anyhow, even if he doesn't want to.

Dr. A.:   Did you hear that Mrs. C.? Bill thinks he should be made to apologize.

Tim: You should beat him till he apologizes. [Group laughs.]

Dr. A.:   The other question is about those who think the parents should apologize. Can you give the reasons for that? [Note that even though Dr. A. has been attempting to arrange for the children to be responsible for their own apologies, he assumes that those who favor apologies by parents have some good reasons. Further, he respects their right to equal time.]

Mrs. R.:   Well, if you're the parent and you raised him, then you should do it. The other parent may cool down a lot faster and not hold it against him so long.

Dr. A.:   So you think its a way of protecting the child.

Mrs. U.:   Many parents don't care what their kids are doing, and they don't let the kids know it's important to apologize.

Mrs. W.:   It's also important to set a good example.

At this point most of the parents are nodding in agreement with the three mothers who first spoke and in disagreement with Dr. A's original prejudice. Dr. A. has always insisted that one reason parents' groups are valuable is that collectively the parents not only make better sense than a single parent but also often make better sense than a single professional. Will he now have the flexible courage of his conviction?

Dr. A.:   I really like what I'm hearing. You're saying that apologizing for your child is a way of protecting him, and it's also a way of setting a good example, teaching him that apologies are important.

Mrs. W.:   (*interrupts*) You mean overprotection?

Dr. A.:   No. I don't mean overprotection—protection from excessive
          social pressure; that can't hurt. It's a normal function for a parent
          to protect a child. The other things you haven't said explicitly in
          words, but you have implied it, is that a child's behavior is a joint
          responsibility of the child and parent. It is the parent and kid
          working together to keep this good behavior. If the kid is not
          behaving, it's kind of like you are both responsible—mostly the
          kid, but somewhat the parent, because you need to be involved in
          that, you need to care about how he is behaving. I think that is a
          pretty good idea, I kind of like that. When I originally asked the
          question, "Why should you apologize for your child's behavior?" I
          was pretty negative about that, but you have convinced me it's
          really a pretty good idea.

Mrs. L.: As a parent, you're really kind of saying to the child, "I'm not
          going to accept that kind of behavior."

Dr. A.:   There's also an element here of one human being stating to
          another that someone has been hurt and deserves recognition of
          that hurt. Well, you've all taught me something today. [The new
          insight is still compatible with the child's being responsible to
          apologize, and Dr. A. feels that this responsibility has not been
          adequately explored, so he turns again to the children.] What
          about this idea that you don't want to apologize? You've hurt
          somebody, and you really should say you're sorry and apologize.
          You've taken something that doesn't belong to you, or you've
          called them a bad name. [Scott's hand up.] OK, Scott, what do
          you think?

Scott: You should give him back what you took. [Many parents voice
          approval of Scott's statement.]

Dr. A.:   Good. You should have to replace what you've taken or any dam-
          age you've done, or work it off.

Mrs. N.: Mother may have to pay originally, but then the child can pay her
          back. [Other parents nod.]

Dr. A.:   It looks like there is something to it. All the parents can't be
          wrong. Let's talk about what Tim said: if a kid should be beaten
          till he says he's sorry. Scott, what was your idea about that?

Scott: Tell the other kid's mom.

Dr. A.:   You should tell the other kid's mom?

Scott: Tell her you're sorry.

Dr. A.:   If a kid does something wrong to another kid, he should apologize to the other kid's parent instead of to the kid?

Scott: He could beat you up.

How would you respond to Scott's bizarre comment? Apparently Scott feels it would be safer to contact the other child's parent with an apology than to approach the offended child directly. Contained within Scott's strange precaution is an implied object lesson that Dr. A. makes explicit before returning to the important issue of passive-aggressiveness:

Dr. A.:   Yes. Anybody could beat you up if you did something wrong to him. [This reflection settles for the preconventional level of morality at which Scott seems to be operating.] What do you think the parents should do if the kid does something wrong and he won't apologize, even though the parents explain what he did wrong?

Tricia: You could take away their privileges until they do it.

Dr. A.:   OK, that sounds like a good idea.

Mrs. R.:   (*impatiently*) I think you should take the child by the hand and go apologize! I don't have to take their privileges away. He'll stand there till he apologizes!

Dr. A.:   You'll just physically hold him there till he apologizes?

Two mothers: Yes!

Dr. A.:   Oh, you're saying that the parent needs to take charge, take control of that situation.

Mrs. W.:   I think if you do that, you are showing the kid the right thing to do.

Dr. A.:   That's an excellent point. And you are also setting an example of caring. OK, what comes next?

Scott: Feedback!

Part III
Training Group Leaders

26
Supervision after an Easy Group

In the training process for group leadership, Dr. A first demonstrates for several groups with the trainee in attendance. Then the trainee takes the lead while Dr. A kibbitzes as cotherapist and takes notes and/or tapes for postgroup supervisory critique. Gradually Dr. A's role phases into mainly note taking and taping. Finally, the trainee takes the group alone and tapes it for supervisory critique. This and the following two chapters are transcripts of supervisory sessions going over tapes and notes of parents' groups that child psychiatry fellows led. The tape that Dr. A. and Dr. N. are listening to is transcribed in italics. After introductions, Dr. N. had asked the parents how the children had been the past week.

Dr. A.: That's always a good standby if there is not some obvious theme that has come up in the first segment of group and if some parent doesn't have some pressing thing that they're obviously eager to get started on. Today it didn't seem as if anyone had anything pressing, and it seemed as if they needed some direction, which you gave them.

> Mr. Q.: *Dana rejects responsibility. She usually hates coming here. We can predict that on Wednesdays she'll give us a hard time. She's kind of introverted, and I think she doesn't like the group. I think it is the pressure of reporting in the group.*

> Mrs. H.: *Tony seems to be getting into his assignments. He even seems to be picking up on the example of our foster daughter who is responsible for cleaning up after herself. He seems to like something new and different and seems to take an interest in a constructive way.*

Dr. A.: At this point you could have explored the topic of novelty and maintaining the interest of the child, but it is not really wrong that you didn't. Your approach through much of this group was more of a laissez-faire, one that is not my style, but it worked well with this group of parents, who were fairly verbal and were able to relate to each other's problems.

Dr. N.: Mr. Q. turned the topic to the parents' side of the problem.

> Mr. Q.: *I'm not able to not respond. She catches me off guard and tricks me into going back to my old tricks of yelling or nagging at her or pressuring her. I feel like I am losing control and going back into my old pattern, where she forces me to watch her and have to pay attention to her instead of doing jobs around the house. When she's behaving, it's hard to give her attention and not work on the house, even though I know I should. Just seeing the jobs that need to be done bothers me.*

Dr. A.: At this point, you did something very useful in the group process: you picked up on the feeling behind Mr. Q.'s ventilation and in particular that aspect of the feeling that you knew from other sources was in common with other members of the group. You explicitly verbalized and identified the feeling of frustration. The validity of that move was corroborated by the fact that Mrs. E., who up to this point had been silent, with a rather discouraged look on her face, perked up and ventilated some of her frustration and discouragement, with the result of being able to end on a philosophically upbeat note.

> Mrs. E.: *Yes, we've been very discouraged about Dale. It seems as if nothing we do helps. He seems so proud of reporting that this week he had lied every day. [His assignment was to keep from lying the previous week.] One thing though, he did tell the truth about lying all week. That's one thing he was truthful about.*

Dr. A.: Here's one missed opportunity that I didn't think of at the time myself. In retrospect, I wish we had said something like, "That's a very useful thought, Mrs. E.; I wish I had thought of that. If we had pointed out to Dale the positive aspect of what he had done right there in the group—telling the truth about lying—we might have helped start him off on the right foot. It would have been kind of forcing him to do something right—catching him being good. After all, he could have lied about lying, and you're very correct that we should pay attention to even this much truthfulness. That would also have taken the wind out of his sails if he was bragging about 100 percent lying, which, of course, we don't want to reinforce by paying attention to it."

Unfortunately, Mrs. H. filled the vacuum left by our nonintervention with her good-intentioned but inept, confused, superior-sounding attempt to talk about the need for both reward and punishment. To that effort of hers, you replied with a move that I basically agree with; I don't think we should let someone continue with something that another parent would see as naive or destructive or a put-down, but I don't understand the particular form your intervention took. You said, "Children like this usually respond better to positive reinforcement than punishment." That's true, but it sounded to me like you were telling her she was wrong, which also could have been true, but maybe there was a more constructive way of stating it.

Dr. N.: What I was trying to deal with here was her misguided advocacy of paradoxical intention: her suggestion that since Dale didn't seem to respond in a normal way to reward, Mrs. E. should try punishing him for doing the right thing.

Dr. A.: Oh, I missed that. I didn't realize she was on that track. Perhaps you could have capitalized on it in a way that was complimentary to Mrs. H., something like, "I think you're right, Mrs. H., that Dale doesn't respond to reward and punishment in the usual way, and that, of course, is one of the things that makes him so frustrating to Mrs. E.—that when she rewards him, he reacts as if he's been punished, and when she punishes him he acts as if he has been rewarded." This would formulate what you thought Mrs. H. was groping for and state it in such a way that she would probably agree with it and could appear to be empathic to Mrs. E. rather than merely giving cheap advice from a smarter-than-thou stance. This would have helped to establish rapport between the two mothers.

Since Mrs. H. did not seem to be able to formulate a constructive plan based on paradoxical intention or therapeutic double bind, it would have been OK for you to suggest one, such as, "Maybe the way to handle Dale's opposition is to plan on having him tell the truth on Tuesday, Thursday, and Saturday, and to lie on Monday, Wednesday, Friday, and Sunday. Then even if he lies all the time, it would be a partial success. If he reverses the days, he would still be telling the truth half the time." By interspersing truth and lie days, he'll have something to compare the truth with to try to get a feel of what it is like to tell the truth.

Dr. N.: I guess I just wasn't quick enough tuning in to the problem. I didn't quite know what to do with it.

Dr. A.: Of course, what I am saying is with twenty-twenty hindsight; it's always easier to quarterback after the game's over. I miss plenty of those opportunities, too.

> Mrs. E.: *I never have trouble with Dale when he's told absolutely to do something or not do something. It's just that he won't do the right thing on his own. He has to be told every little thing exactly; then he does it.*

> Dr. N.: *You've really had some discouraging days.*

Dr. A.: This was a useful bit of empathizing. It put the group back on an empathic channel after the stress between Mrs. H. and Mrs. E.

> Mr. Q.: *I wish Dana would understand my need for some reinforcement. If I don't get some reinforcement, it gets to me. I have to know that what I'm doing has some payoff.*

Dr. A.: Mr. Q. is here providing the first opportunity of exploring the problem of parents' need to have approval from their children, but it is not yet clear that that is what he is working on, and I agree with your delay until he provides a little more material, as he does shortly.

> Mrs. C.: *I'm never able to get away from George. It's like I'm trapped with him. He just clings with me, and he's everywhere that I am. I invent a reason to go shopping to get away from him.*

> Mrs. Q.: *When I'm away from Dana for a while, then I can return and be much more stable rather than jump on her when I shouldn't. I think it is really good for the parents to get away from the kids for a while.*

> Mr. Q.: *I like to have constructive interaction, but I need to do other things sometimes, too. But it seems as if the kid*

reads that as rejection, if you don't spend 100 percent of your time with them. It isn't that I don't love them, but I have other things I have to do, too.

Dr. N.: *Do you ever say, "I need an hour to do this; then I'll do what you want me too"?*

Dr. A.: There is not really anything wrong with this kind of practical suggestion, but it seems as if you missed the opportunity for something more telling. By this time, I think you've had enough evidence that Mr. Q. needs his child's approval to feel like a good parent. This is such an important issue that whenever you see it presented clearly, you need to give it high priority.

Mrs. Q.: *We've done that kind of thing, but every five seconds she keeps asking "When will you be done? How much longer?"*

Dr. A.: Mrs. Q.'s response shows the pitfall of rushing in with a concrete suggestion before finding out what they have already tried. Fortunately, you did not really advise them to do that; you asked them whether they had tried it, presumably to find out what the reaction was or how it worked out. Now you need to follow up with further exploration: for example, as to whether they had taught her how to watch the hands of a clock. Remember, though, for a child of this age, it looks as though the hands never move. You need to give her some other time measurement device, such as having her work a puzzle and come back to see how far the hands had moved, so she could understand that for the hands to move a certain distance is the same amount of time as it takes to work her puzzle.

An even better idea, though, would have been to pick up on the bottomless pit aspect of the child's demand for attention and time. The bottomless pit phenomenon and the need to set limits on the amount of time a parent can give, give it freely, and then not feel guilty would lead naturally into the underlying theme about the parents' feeling of need for the child's approval. Mr. Q. keeps knocking on the door with that problem.

Mr. Q.: *If I can get Dana to realize that I need her to get things done and feel some success myself, I think things would be a lot better.*

Dr. N.: *You need to feel in charge. The kids are more confident and secure when the kid feels the parent is in charge.*

Dr. N.: *(to Dr. A.)* That was my attempt to speak to the need-for-approval problem. I don't think it was a very effective way of doing it. What else could I have said?

Dr. A.: I think you were on the right track, but you didn't verbalize the key issue here, which was timing. Mr. Q. keeps wanting some kind of reassurance from Dana now, which you are implying that he can get eventually in the future because when Dana grows up, she will appreciate his being firm now. It's premature for him to expect that kind of feedback now. You could have used an analogy of investing for future payback. Your failure to mention the timing issue at all leaves the focus on current payback.

> Mrs. Q.: *If the kids feel more confident and secure, why do they fight it and complain so much?*

> Mr. Q.: *I don't want good behavior by intimidation. I don't want Dana to be afraid of me, just to respect me and behave because it's the right thing.*

Dr. A.: Here it would be a good thing to talk about how parents need to love children enough to make them do the right thing even though it makes them feel like heels, even when it makes the parent feel like a meanie. You need to reinterpret the heavy role as being a good father rather than as being an intimidating martinet.
[Now Dr. A. and Dr. N. abandon the tape and rely on memory and notes that Dr. A. had taken.]

Mrs. W. mentioned something about a lot of tears, but I didn't recall what that was all about.

Dr. N.: They started saying that they had wanted their child to be happy all the time. They don't know why she's not happy; that they have all the adult things to worry about, like bills, and they expect her to be happy. It disturbs them that she is not happy any of the time. She bursts into tears a lot.

There were several ways to go with that. I wanted to say that possibly medication would make a child more prone to tearful outbursts, but also I wanted to point out that childhood is not an idyllic paradise like adults want to remember it, that children have a great deal of fears and worries that adults probably don't appreciate. I think a parent shouldn't expect a child to be happy all the time or feel that it is their duty to make them happy all the time. I tried to bring that out. I wanted them to talk it out.

Dr. A.: I agree with you that childhood is a painful experience. The better childhood you have, the worse it might seem because you can remember it better. If it's too bad, you repress it all and can't remember it.

Dr. N.: I was kind of wondering about Mrs. Q.'s childhood because she said she couldn't remember it before age thirteen. It must have been pretty bad.

Dr. A.: It's pretty routine to repress most of your childhood; at least that's what I've run into with people, especially those who talk about how much fun it is to be a child. I'm sure they have repressed it. [Laughter between Dr. N. and Dr. A.] OK, so your response to that was to talk about selective forgetting, how tough it is to be a child and how a kid has the right to be unhappy. That's all legitimate stuff to bring out. But there was something else that happened here. Mrs. E. said that *she* hadn't seen a tear from Dale in four years.

Dr. N.: Right . . . I wanted to bring that up, but it got buried under some other stuff. I wanted to talk about why Dale never cried.

Dr. A.: I think I would have picked up on it with some remark like, "Does that worry you that he doesn't cry?" Or ask the others, "What would you think? You're worried about your child crying; would you rather trade places with Mrs. E.? She never sees her son, Dale, cry." Maybe they would have realized how lucky they are having a child who could cry in front of them.

Dr. N.: Right.

Dr. A.: The lack of tears could indicate that he's lost his affect or that he thinks that he has to keep a brave front, be tough. It's hard to tell.
    In regard to selective memory, Mrs. Q. said, "It depends on how you were brought up in the past." That was a very insightful comment. You mentioned about her not remembering anything before age thirteen. She said, "I try to be a little more liberal, like my husband was brought up, but we have some disagreements about how we manage the children."

Dr. N.: That would have been a good time to bring up about "what do you do?"

Dr. A.: Or "How do you resolve differences?" or "Is there a right way?" Then Mr. E. said, "Things that I call the kids down on, my father sometimes says to me afterwards that it's no big deal, that I did the same thing as a kid. I don't remember, but I think, 'Why did he let me get away with it? He shouldn't have.'" This would have been a good time, incidentally, to underscore that: "See, kids really do think limit setting is important. You're miffed at your father for not having limited you."

Dr. N.: But if he's doing it as an adult now, he might disqualify that.

Dr. A.: If he replies, "But I'm an adult now; that's why I appreciate it," you can say, "Would you rather have Dale miffed at you now for ten years and then appreciate for the next sixty years what you did for him, or would you rather give in to him now and have him miffed at you for sixty years?"

Dr. N.: That's a good point.

Dr. A.: He said, "I get to thinking about some of those things Dale does, and I think maybe they're not such a big deal, but they just happen to get on my nerves." What could you have done with that?

Dr. N.: It would have been a good thing to get into how one's mood affects limit setting, and should it affect limiting setting, and how can you get around it affecting limit setting. [Dr. A. nods.]

Dr. A.: Good. Also, what are the parents' rights versus the child's rights? The child has a right for parents not to be capricious and whimsical about the limits they set, but on the other hand parents also have the right to have the headache that they happen to have that day considered. Maybe they ordinarily wouldn't mind the kid pounding on something, but maybe this particular day, he needs to give up his pounding until tomorrow because you happen to have a headache today.

Then Mrs. E. said, "What do you do when the child is running you around in front of company? They don't realize what he's up to, what he's doing, but you do." It might have been interesting to ask her for an example, because it sounds like he's engaged in some kind of sociopathic maneuver or machiavelian plot, and she knows what he's up to. It sounds a little paranoid, but I don't think it is. I think he really does do things. He's an opportunist; we know that. [Dr. N. nods.] But it might be good to get an example.

Dr. N.: Yes. I feel a little protective of Mrs. E. because of her speech difficulty. There were some times when I didn't understand her, and that may have been the times I didn't elaborate when I should have. Perhaps I should demand a little more of her.

Dr. A.: Good self-observation. She also said that "it used to be that I would wait until the company leaves and then deal with the problem. But now I correct him right away in front of the company, and I don't care what they think of me." She got some accolades from Mr. Q. about that. He went on to say that they used to be in the same fix. Anytime they would be in a restaurant, Dana could get away with murder because she knew they wouldn't do anything about it in front of the other people. Mrs. Q. said, "Now I just take her to the bathroom to settle her if she starts acting up."

Dr. N.: That's one place they have made some significant gains; that's one of the problems they came in for.

Dr. A.: The father went on to say, "We even figured out that other people really do respect you more for taking action; that we should have been more embarrassed about letting her get away with it than limit setting. We see the people approve of what we're doing when we try to limit Dana's bad behavior." Then Mrs. H. said, "You are the controlling factor." What was the point of that?

Dr. N.: I think she just meant that parents need to exert control when kids are out of control. That she's forgot that Greg needs external control.

Dr. A.: Then Mrs. E. says Dale can be nice when it's to his advantage. He is good when he's visiting friends. I would have tried to explain to her that he's good when it's fun, naturally. And I might have asked her if he could stay a little longer with those people. Why hasn't she thought of that?

Dr. N.: Yes! I wasn't sure if these were friends or relatives.

Dr. A.: If she wanted to prove what he's like, she should try to get him to stay a week or two. That would give her a breather and one of two things would happen: (1) someone else would have found out what he's really like, and she could then feel vindicated, or (2) he could behave well the whole time and get in the habit of better behavior. Putting it in another way, it would prove to her it's possible. Right now she doesn't believe. One of the problems we are dealing with is that she doesn't really expect him to shape up.

Dr. N.: I think that's a good point. We need to explore that.

Dr. A.: If we prove to her once that he can do it, she might have more expectations.

Dr. N.: I don't think that it is her fault. But some parents think that if their child behaves well for someone else, they are failures as parents. Mrs. E. has had to give up a career except for household duties due to her illness; maybe she really sees that saving Dale is her career, and it's not going well and it lowers her self-esteem.

Dr. A.: Dana had said that she didn't misbehave at school because she's not allowed to act that way.

Dr. N.: And mother said, "What makes you think you can act this way here?"

Dr. A.: That was a good point on mother's part.

Dr. N.: And Dana didn't answer. I just wonder what kind of cues mother gives that makes Dana feel that it's OK to act up at home.

Dr. A.: At this point you could ask the parents, "If she needs a safety valve somewhere—you might want to think twice about this because for some parents it wouldn't be good to say it—would you rather she misbehave at school or at home?" Most parents probably would say "at home" and see it as a positive thing that she behaves well at school. You could say, "Would you rather she misbehaves at home where you can deal with it?" This would help the parents set the expectations of change, that they are not supposed to just accept it. They could see this as positive because it would be much more difficult for them to control what she does at school.

Mrs. E. said she asked Dale why he misbehaves, and he said, "Because I want to." It might have been nice to have asked how the others deal with that sort of arrogant, egocentric thinking. Mr. B.'s response was, "The way they bluff, can you imagine them playing poker?" Maybe a little bit of pride in the kid's ability to bluff. Mr. B. then said that it seems as if a little fuss sets off a big stick of dynamite. Then Mrs. H. said that she thought the kids were smarter—not really smarter but more unpredictable. Then you brought out that if you play by rules, you are more predictable; if you don't follow rules, you are more unpredictable and harder to deal with, naturally. This would have been a good place to explain the phenomenon of requisite variety: how the least predictable person controls an interaction if the other is not prepared. Perhaps the kids need to be shown other ways to control. Mr. H. then said, "I guess it would be the same situation with an irrational, unpredictable adult. What I want to do is raise Greg to be a rational adult." What he was really talking about was modeling. This is a good place to talk about how they were really modeling that for the kids by being rational, predictable adults, even though the kids didn't seem to respond to it or appreciate it at the time. Through modeling and imitation is how the kids learn, which will have a long-term effect.

Dr. N.: All these parents needed to hear that.

27
Supervision around Pitfalls

I n this supervisory session, Dr. N. is relating a parents' group to Dr. A. from memory.

Dr. N.: Mrs. D. [Betty's mother] started off with a plan that we had talked about the last time they were here. Betty would get a star or some kind of special recognition for paying attention to the teacher that day. She needed some immediate feedback. Mrs. D. spoke to the teacher about it, and she had refused to do it. Mrs. D. was rather discouraged because she had expected more cooperation. Although the teacher was excellent in a lot of ways, she said she couldn't show favoritism because all the kids would want it. I said it was kind of sad that the teacher didn't realize that Betty had special needs that the other children didn't have, and I asked the parents if they felt that they had to treat children exactly the same, even when they had different needs.

   Mrs. H. (Bob and Tom's mother) pointed out that she realized her boys had different needs. I pointed out that with children so close in ages, it's easy to treat them exactly alike. I tried to point out that it is more fair to treat children differently than the same. The parents all nodded and seemed agreeable. Then Mrs. D. devised a system where she would give Betty a flower sticker for every day that she was good in school.

Dr. A.: But how did she know Betty was good that day?

Dr. N.: I don't know. I'm a little confused myself on that.

Dr. A.: What she needed was some indication from the teacher. Was the teacher willing to communicate with mother by telephone?

Dr. N.: We didn't explore that, but that's a possibility. Mother said it had worked. I guess she had asked Betty whether she was good and would give her a flower on that basis. But we don't know if it is accurate or not.

Dr. A.: What she might have been doing is reinforcing lying.

Dr. N.: Possibly, but she said it had been working.

Dr. A.: It may have worked in Betty's case because she may be that ingenuous, but in general this is a risky thing to do, to reinforce a verbalization unless the verbalization has intrinsic merit. For example, if you want to reinforce a child's saying "thank you" or reinforce his saying something nice to a playmate, that's fine because the verbalization there is the desired goal in and of itself. But you don't want to reinforce the child saying that he has performed a desired action. What you may end up doing is reinforcing lying.

Dr. N.: That may be true, but Mrs. D. wanted to express her frustration to the group because it was Mrs. K. who had proposed the star for paying attention to the teacher. It had worked for Aaron and had carried over, even when they had stopped.

Mrs. K. reported that Aaron is starting not to cooperate in taking his medication. She has been putting out his pill, expecting him to take it, and he has been dropping in on the floor, losing it. She wanted to know how the H.'s were doing it. I asked Mrs. K. if Aaron recognized the benefit of taking the medication, if he feels he is more able to be in control with the medication. She said that she felt that he did, but she didn't understand why he was not taking his pill. We talked a bit about some payoffs a child may get out of not taking his pill, like an excuse to misbehave or an excuse to be out of control. With a pill, a kid may not have an excuse to be bad. Mr. H. had said that Bob and Tom had done that on occasion.

Dr. A.: What was your idea in bringing this out? I agree that there are various reasons like that, but why bring it out now?

Dr. N.: My eventual point was, "It is very admirable that you are trying to encourage independence, but the price of that is you have to be able to accept him not following through—like whether you are willing to let them dress themselves and put their T-shirt on backwards. You have to be willing to tolerate that." I said, "You may be willing to tolerate him not taking his medication, or you may feel that this is one thing you are not going to give him responsibility for."

Dr. A.:　It's too important to leave it up to him?

Dr. N.:　Right. I said, "It is up to you to decide whether independence is more important than taking the pill." Then Mrs. H. said there were times when the boys wouldn't take it, and she had to force it down them. Now that they are older, they take it themselves. I pointed out that at age six, Aaron is probably a little young to be taking his own medication, but it was up to parents to decide how much independence they would encourage and what the trade-off would be.

Dr. A.:　There is another issue here: is the issue of the pill taking getting sucked into control struggles? I can see that happening very easily with Aaron because he is oppositional. It gets sucked into the struggle two ways: One is, "By golly, you little rat, I'm going to make sure you take this whether you like it or not, and you're not going to get away with spitting it out or refusing to take it." The second way is, "I'm going to put this pill in you because then you will behave, and that's my way of controlling you, through this chemical means." Both of those are pitfalls. It's very important for parents to be aware and not get sucked into these kinds of control struggles. Medication should be seen as something that is good for the kid, not something that helps the parents to control him and not something as a matter of parental pride. They need to be able to take the attitude, "I care enough about you to make sure you get this medicine, which is going to help you, make it easier for you to control yourself, to behave." The emphasis should be on the child controlling himself and the parent supporting that by aiding the child in controlling himself, to be more autonomous.

Dr. N.:　That was the reason why I pointed out that a child may have his own reasons for wanting to behave or not behave independently of the medication. I think Mrs. K. tends to feel the pill is magic; that when he takes his pill, he's a perfectly behaved child and when he doesn't, he's totally unmanageable. I wanted to point out that he has volitional control to a large degree, that it's not just the magic of a pill. It seemed to be a revelation to Mrs. K. that he could choose, or not choose, to behave.

Dr. A.:　Even with the pill, he could still misbehave.

Dr. N.:　Right. Mrs. K. even talked about how she knows he didn't take the pill because he was so wild that day.

Dr. A.: That kind of assumes that the child will never act bad unless it is the illness that's doing it.

Dr. N.: Then Mrs. H. brought up how she was involved in a power struggle with her son. We talked about how hard it is to be the meanie, how hard it is to enforce rules and stay calm and not get involved in the power struggle; that it really does work. I really appreciated Mrs. H.'s input. She got tears in her eyes, and she said she realized how far they had come. Mrs. M. brought up how her son, Dick, really won the battle. He managed to get two school teachers to escort him out to home.

Dr. A.: It sounds like the theme here is that you can't depend on school personnel to do things for your kid. They will get sucked into power struggles with him, and they won't meet his special needs. That's a good topic to get into: how to get from the school what you need for your kid and how you help your kid survive even though he's not being provided with what you think he needs.

Dr. N.: We didn't get into that specifically. I did praise Mrs. D. for making up a compensatory system for Betty. We did talk about long-term rewards versus short-term rewards. Mrs. M. and Mrs. D. did talk about their dissatisfaction with the school.

Dr. A.: Some parents bring teachers in for group, and that may be a possibility for this family.

Dr. N.: I think the group was pretty good, all in all, except for the new parents, who didn't participate.

Dr. A.: What are some ways you could have drawn them into it?

Dr. N.: It seemed like the time was moving so fast. They seemed to be paying very close attention.

Dr. A.: They were nonverbally participating?

Dr. N.: They seemed like they were with us.

Dr. A.: What about some time when they were nodding? That would have been a good opportunity to say their name and either verbalize their agreement—"It looks like you've had the same experience"—or ask them to comment. Ordinarily a new parent is given the floor early in the group. Usually we have to watch to keep a new parent from taking things over. But occasionally we need to take the opposite tack. The important thing is to maintain a balance between the new parents and the veterans.

28
Supervision after a Difficult Group

Occasionally a group taxes all the assertiveness and expertise the leader can muster. The most common cause of a difficult group is an aggressively destructive, dominant person who seems insensitive to the ordinary cues for constructive group work. Most parents, even if exasperated and hostile (even rejecting) initially, soon pick up cues from staff and other parents to work constructively and hopefully. However, an occasional rejecting parent continues hostile to the child even after repeated group contacts. Dr. M.'s struggles to limit the destructiveness of one such mother are discussed in the following supervision transcript. Dr. M. and Dr. A. start out listening to the tape of parents' group, which appears in italics.

> Dr. M.: *We have several new families here today, so why don't one of the veterans tell them what goes on in the group.*

> Mrs. K.: *I'm Cynthia K. We get together to air off so you know you're not alone, to get support or ideas. Basically, I think it is to air out what you want to say, bad or good, about your child.*

> Dr. M.: *If a parent faces the same problem, they can learn from how the other parent solved the problem.*

Dr. A.: It's good that you pointed out another option for the group, because otherwise they set it up as a kind of a bitch session. You could have even gone down the list of options.

Dr. M.: I did mention other options later.

Dr. A.: OK. Good.

> Dr. M.: *We can use the group in any way we want, education or airing off or other things. We have about forty-five*

minutes, and then we rejoin the kids. The group can be educationally oriented, or I can present a minilecture.

Dr. A.: I thought your first intervention—where you said it can also be educational—that was good. But I think in succeeding statements you need to explain what you mean by that rather than just using the same words over again. And I think I would have chosen as an example of education not that you would give minilectures (you could have added that on) but the idea that maybe they can give each other ideas, about how they try things that might work and things that didn't work, what they have learned from their mistakes, what they've learned from their successes, and support and help each other. And then maybe jokingly add, "Maybe I'll even be able to help you." Whenever you bring yourself into it, I think you need to qualify it as to the limitations because most of these people will come with the idea that the professional is the one who is going to give the answers. And the idea of group is that they can give each other answers or at least help each other clarify the problems better than we could one to one.

Dr. M.: Yes, I see. Then in the middle of the discussion, Mrs. K. suddenly asked for advice about Sean.

Mrs. K.: *Didn't Dr. A. say before we came in that we were going to speak on what Sean had done? [Mrs. K. had begun castigating Sean in front of the whole group while the parents and children were together, and Dr. A. had suggested that her complaints be delayed to parents' group.] He was supposed to go to bed on time, and then at the end of the week we would reinforce him with Dairy Queen. When he received the money he had earned from someone else, he spent it on ice cream. But it was like on Monday, so the week was half over with. But he really hadn't earned it, going to bed like he chose in his project. He doesn't do anything. I make him dress or otherwise he would go to school late. He doesn't do anything.*

Mrs. P.: (interrupts) *He's not motivated.*

Mrs. K.: (nods) *He's not motivated at all. [She continues for five or ten minutes, blaming, complaining, and finding fault with Sean.]*

Dr. A.: Stop it right there because she has strayed from a clearly stated problem: "What do we do about a leak in the system?" [In a behavior modification paradigm, he gets the reward in some other way. There's a leak in the system.] She veers off from that to a kind of general platitudinal impugnment of his character, his lack of motivation. She said he's not motivated, but she skipped over the reason he isn't motivated, which is that he doesn't have to work for the reward. You need to stop her right there and say, "What do you think is the reason he's not motivated?" And she'll probably say, "Well, that's just the way he is." Then you could say, "Well, you told me the reason he's not motivated when you first started out. Did the rest of you hear it?" And just pull the others in: "Would you tell Mrs. K. what the reason is that Sean is not motivated? She gave us the reason." I'm sure that somebody would quickly figure out what it is you want, and they would say, "Sure, he gets his reward without working for it. That's why he's not motivated." Of course, if they don't get it, you can state it or give a clue, like, "Could the fact that he got the reward without working have anything to do with it?"

Dr. M.: I struggled to find a good opportunity to stop her.

Dr. A.: She'll never give you a good opportunity. You have to make an opportunity.

Dr. M.: She has a lot of material.

Dr. A.: There are several ways to approach somebody that's on a filibuster. One is that you decide on something that you want to bring the subject back to, and you wait for them to say something that's tangential to it, something that can be related in any way, and sooner or later they'll give you a chance. Somebody like this, talking at that pace and flitting around, sooner or later is going to hit on a subject that is related to it. You're all prepared, you're alert for that, to be able to snatch it in midair and say, "That reminds me of what you said before," or, "That comes back to the point you first made. I wonder what the other parents think about that point." Or, as in this case, "You say he's unmotivated; well, we have the answer for that; you gave us the answer."

Another approach is just to say, "Well, maybe we should give the other parents a chance to talk," or, "I'd like to know what the other parents think about it." Sometimes if you're really feeling strongly that somebody is being destructive, as she sometimes gets to be, you just need to say, "We're trying to keep this on a constructive note. Everyone here, I'm sure, has heard all kinds of horror stories about how bad their kid is at times, but we're trying to figure out how to improve that. Now let's take the problem you're presenting and figure out how you can improve it. Maybe the others have some ideas"—again turning it to the others. You have to limit her because she can't limit herself or the child. Like billiard balls, your limit setting will transfer the momentum, and she will be better able to limit her child's behavior.

Dr. M.: Do you think I could have stopped her when she mentioned letting off air in the beginning? Maybe that was permission to let off air.

Dr. A.: You mean that she was asking if it was OK to just let off steam? Well, that's a thought. One of the purposes of the group is to ventilate. So that was OK. You want to be careful that somebody like this doesn't train you to shoot from the hip too quickly because you know from past experience with her that she is going to do this sort of thing. You need to look for the opportunity to do what she fails to do with her son: catch her doing the right thing and reinforce her for it. You have to be alert for her to change in a constructive direction. You had her doing the right thing for a minute. You had her telling about the reinforcement paradigm. If you can catch her in that and reinforce her, she might escalate constructiveness. You don't want to keep swatting her down unnecessarily.

> Mrs. K.: *I was surprised this weekend. He was behaving terribly. He usually wants to go to his father's, but this time he didn't. I let him decide on his own what he wanted to do. He just called his father and told him that he wasn't going to go this weekend.*

Dr. M.: The reason why I let her talk so long was that she brings up a lot of things the others could concentrate on. I was waiting for someone to pick up on something.

Dr. A.: It's all right to let her go for a few minutes until somebody does pick up on it, but if they don't, you could say, "I wonder if somebody else has a similar experience?" Pick something that you can feel pretty confident is a common problem. After someone speaks for so long, some of the others may start tuning out. So you should repeat what it is you are asking about: "Has anybody else had the experience of telling the kid what to do, and then she wanders off and does something else?" But it's OK to let it go for a little while. The others may not be ready to talk yet. They may need the time to formulate what they want to say. A person like this in the group can kind of get the ball rolling.

> *Mrs. V.:*   *That reminds me how Bob came in the other day dragging his kite behind him. We had just bought a kite; he had been behaving better. He was learning how to fly a kite, and way back in February he had got his first kite and it had been too cold on Saturdays to fly it.*

Dr. A.:   I would have asked her if she had made it clear to him that she had got the kite because he had been behaving well. I'm wondering how much she reinforces his improved behavior. She's obviously pleased with him, but I wonder how much she pounces on the opportunity to have a pleasant interaction.

Dr. M.:   I thought maybe we could summarize the progress of each child and their parent in the group.

Dr. A.:   That's a good idea. We probably should do more of that. So many of the parents tend to focus on the negative that they don't notice what is going well.

Dr. M.:   I thought I'd let the parents bring up the problem with the kids when we got back together.

Dr. A.:   One thing you have to be careful of is not seeming to set up a conspiracy with the parents, to finger a kid in the group when you get back with the kids. I think you came close to doing that today. You need to keep things very general and identify with the kids. Your attitude should be something like, "Here is something that the parents talked about that you kids would be interested in discussing," rather than, "Here is something the parents thought you kids should be told." The latter seems to identify as an agent of the parent. Of course, my paraphrasing exaggerates what you did for the sake of making the point, but the subtle difference is crucial. I heard a discussion die aborning once when the leader confronted the kids with something like "One thing the parents talked about was how much you kids cuss. Who in here cusses?" The kids immediately clammed up, but I'm sure would have responded nicely to "The parents talked about cussing. Who can tell me what cussing is?"

On the other hand, I don't think it's wrong to call on a certain kid to say, "Here's something you seem to have a problem with." Your evidence for saying that would be from something the child said in the group, not what the parents told you about the child. It could best be done with a couple of kids at the same time: for example, "Bob and Jeff, you both said something earlier when you reported about how you both planned your goal real well, but it didn't seem to work." You can name certain kids that way. It just makes them feel like you paid attention to what they've said. They'll be pleased that you noticed them.

Dr. M.: In one situation I tried to find a reason for the behavior and tried to question the child about it, but it didn't seem to work. How could I have done that better?

Dr. A.: One important thing is language, to use words the kids can understand, getting rid of jargon or fancy words. The other point is just having the experience to know immediately five different reasons and remembering them. It's just a matter of being exposed to a lot of patients and developing a repertoire. You'll have it with time.

29
Conclusion and Summary

None of the components of the multifamily sandwich group is original—only the particular synthesis, integration, and structure are. That the whole is greater than the sum of the parts is attested to by observation of either the group or group videotapes. The children's response is such that some observers challenge whether the children seen really have valid behavioral diagnoses. Yet over 75 percent meet DSM-III criteria for attention deficit disorder with hyperactivity or conduct disorder or both, including research criterion scores on the Conners and Davids hyperkinetic scales rated by teachers and parents. Some of the children were being considered for inpatient or residential treatment at the time of referral to the group. Most children and their parents show definite improvement by the third time in attendance. If there is no improvement by the fourth time, additional or alternate therapy (such as medication, individual psychotherapy, or residential treatment) is recommended.

Unfortunately, outcome assessment at this point is essentially anecdotal. On telephone follow-up questionnaires of 36 families, 93 percent felt that the group had been helpful and that the child remained improved. The positive responses and narrative comments suggested that whatever benefits accrued were a result of simultaneously paying attention to (1) the child's needs (success experience, self-esteem, peer relations, and social skills); (2) the parents' needs (empathy, peer support, instrumental knowledge, and hope); and (3) the needs of the parent-child relationship (mutual respect, rights, duties, realization of loving commitment, and tolerance for feelings and imperfections). A more scientifically rigorous examination of group effectiveness is needed.

Summary Review

This multifamily parent-child group treatment is structured into a one-and-three-quarter-hour time sandwich. Separate simultaneous parents' and children's groups are sandwiched between two parent-child sessions.

The first combined parent-child segment, lasting ten to fifteen minutes, includes introductions, reports by the children of their projects picked the previous time, and a short quiz on the importance of planning. At each step, the children are asked to remember what comes next. They are also asked to remember the three parts of the report in proper order: goal ("what you were going to do"), plan ("how you were going to remember to do it"), and score ("how well you did"). The score must be in numbers, such as "five out of seven days" or "13 out of 19 chances."

The children's activity group, lasting forty to fifty minutes, includes a short initial planning session and some group activities calculated to improve sensorimotor integration, cooperative teamwork and other social skills, peer relations, and self-image as a success. Success is defined as improving one's own performance and helping another to improve. The activities range from the strenuous (obstacle courses or running games) to sedate table activities (form boards or group painting). Competitiveness is downplayed; but when it crops up, a discussion is focused on resolving it. The children are allowed some choice of activity within the bounds of constructiveness, but once the group decides by majority vote, all members are expected to carry through the activity to the end. Sometimes political compromise in the planning session allows all the children to have some time on their own favorite activity.

The parents' group lasts forty to fifty minutes, simultaneous with the children's group. It includes the introduction of parents, mutual support, sharing, self-help, witnessing, education and explanation, and minilectures by the professional leader. Topics may include behavioral management (with mutual critique of management paradigms), medication, diagnosis, dealing with school, and titrating protectiveness, directiveness, worry, punishment, indulgence, and other parental impulses. Parents' group is the least structured part of the whole group. The leader should feel free to range, as circumstances warrant, from group psychotherapist through facilitator to educator or even limit setter.

The last combined parent-child segment lasts thirty to forty-five minutes. It includes four sections: (1) a report by the children on their activities, with discussion of how they specifically benefitted; (2) a Socratic discussion with the children on some topic from parents' group; (3) feedback on star charts; and (4) picking of a new project for the coming week. Here again the children are asked at each step to remember what comes next.

The Socratic discussion is the most challenging part of the whole group. It involves simultaneous programming of two sets of people: the children who are interacting and the parents who are listening. The children are gently guided to express constructive ideas and admit problems, and are reinforced for this. The listening parents are thereby programmed to expect sensible, constructive ideas from their children and shown how to elicit and reinforce them. To prevent defensiveness by the children, it is important not to confront: for example, not to say, "Your parents said a lot of kids lie." Rather, an abstract or third person introduction safely removes the topic to a temporarily impersonal distance: for example, say, "One of the things the parents talked about was lying. Who can tell what a lie is? . . . Why would a kid lie? . . . What are some of the reasons?" With the latter approach, the children soon volunteer the reasons they "used to lie."

Star-chart feedback not only has a direct effect on the children's group behavior and performance and gives them a taste of public recognition for success, but also teaches and instigates the parents to use a chart at home. The idea of tracking a specific behavior on a calendar-like table may seem simple and obvious, but most parents do not think of trying it until they see its impact on their child in the group. A dozen or so relevant behaviors are about right for the group star chart.

Project picking is one of the most important parts of group. It provides the continuity from one group to the next and helps generalize the group improvement and success feeling to the rest of the child's life. As much as possible, the goal and plan need to come from the child, but it is alright for children to ask their parents or other group members for ideas from which to choose. Children who try to bite off too big a goal—or too vague and general a goal—need to be gently but firmly limited to a manageable, specific goal. The plan should be something under the child's control. Plans for the parent to remind the child should be discouraged. Plans involving a reward from the parent need to be willingly confirmed by the parent to be allowed. This is the last part of group, and the leader should strive to end on an optimistic note of anticipated responsibility and success by the child with reasonable support by the parents.

Notes

1. C.K. Conners, "A teacher rating scale for use in drug studies with children," *Am. J. Psychiatry* 126 (1969):884–888.

2. A. Davids, "An objective instrument for assessing hyperkinesis in children," *J. Learn. Disabil.* 4 (1971):499–401.

Index

About the Authors

L. Eugene Arnold, M.Ed., M.D., is professor of psychiatry and pediatrics at The Ohio State University, where he is also director of the division of child psychiatry. With a background in liberal arts from St. Charles College, he received his B.S. from the University of Dayton, his M.Ed. from Johns Hopkins University, and his M.D. from The Ohio State University. He interned at the University of Oregon Hospitals and completed residencies at Johns Hopkins University Hospital in psychiatry and child psychiatry. He is executive secretary of The Psychiatric Research Foundation of Columbus and is past chairman of the OSU Bio-Medical Sciences Human Subjects Review Committee. He has written over a hundred contributions to the literature on child mental health and is editor and major contributor to *Helping Parents to Help Their Children* (Brunner Mazel, 1978), *Preventing Adolescent Alienation: An Interprofessional Approach* (Lexington Books, 1983), and *Parents, Children, and Change* (Lexington Books, 1985). He is author of *Parents' Survival Handbook* (Sunbury, Oh.: LAMMP, 1983).

Donna G. Estreicher received her Ph.D. in developmental psychology at The Ohio State University, where she completed an internship at the Nisonger Center. Her special interest has been families of children with developmental disorders; she developed a special approach to include a handicapped child in family therapy. Her clinical experience includes a variety of settings—a children's hospital, a psychiatric clinic, and county mental retardation programs. She has served as guest lecturer at The Ohio State University and has led numerous parents' groups in the community.

Contributor **Katherine S. Sheridan** received her B.S. in allied medical professions, occupational therapy, at The Ohio State University. She specializes in child and adolescent psychiatric occupational therapy, working in both inpatient and outpatient groups. Her current focus is to develop a comprehensive outpatient occupational therapy program.